Essentials of Food Science and Nutrition

Essentials of Food Science and Nutrition

Theo Graham

Callisto Reference

www.callistoreference.com

Callisto Reference,
118-35 Queens Blvd., Suite 400,
Forest Hills, NY 11375, USA

Visit us on the World Wide Web at:
www.callistoreference.com

ISBN: 978-1-64116-630-0 (Hardback)

Cataloging-in-Publication Data

Essentials of food science and nutrition / Theo Graham.
p. cm.
Includes bibliographical references and index.
ISBN 978-1-64116-630-0
1. Food. 2. Food science. 3. Nutrition. 4. Gastronomy. 5. Diet. 6. Cooking. I. Graham, Theo.

TX357 .E77 2022
641.3--dc23

Table of Contents

	Preface	**VII**
Chapter 1	**Food Science and Technology**	**1**
	• Food Science	1
	• Food Technology	3
Chapter 2	**Understanding Nutrition**	**9**
	• Human Nutrition	13
	• Sports Nutrition	26
	• Malnutrition	31
Chapter 3	**Essential Nutrients**	**44**
	• Carbohydrate	44
	• Protein	63
	• Fat	107
	• Vitamin	142
	• Mineral	151
Chapter 4	**Food Supplements**	**155**
	• Fish Oil	157
	• Lactagen	162
	• L-theanine	163
	• Ginkgo Biloba	166
Chapter 5	**Food Additives**	**168**
	• Anticaking Agent	173
	• Food Coloring	175
	• Flour Treatment Agent	177
	• Humectant	179
	• Sugar Substitute	180
	• Thickening Agent	187

Chapter 6 **Allied Aspects of Food Science and Nutrition** **193**
- Food Safety 193
- Food Preservation 194
- Food Chemistry 216
- Food Biotechnology 219
- Food Fortification 221
- Food Microbiology 222
- Food Fermentation 235

Permissions

Index

Preface

The branch of science, which deals with the study of food as well as the fundamental phenomena that are directly linked to its production, is known as food science. It makes use of biological and physical sciences as well as engineering to study the principles behind food processing, the causes of deterioration and the nature of foods. There are various fields which contribute knowledge to food science such as physiology, biochemistry, chemistry, physics and microbiology. Food chemistry, food engineering, food microbiology and food preservation are some of the sub-disciplines of this field. Food chemistry studies the various chemical activities and interactions which take place between the varied non-biological and biological constituents of food. This book provides comprehensive insights into the field of nutrition and food science. It presents researches and studies performed by experts across the globe. Those in search of information to further their knowledge will be greatly assisted by this book.

A short introduction to every chapter is written below to provide an overview of the content of the book:

Chapter 1 - The branch of science which deals with the study of the chemical, physical and biological makeup of food is known as food science. Food technology is involved in the study of the fundamental phenomena which are connected to the production of food products as well as their properties. This is an introductory chapter which will introduce briefly all the significant aspects of food science and technology.; **Chapter 2** - The science of interpreting the interactions between nutrients and other materials in food with respect to the growth, health and disease in an organism is known as nutrition. Some of the sub-disciplines within nutrition are malnutrition and sports nutrition. The chapter closely examines these key concepts of nutrition to provide an extensive understanding of the subject.; **Chapter 3** - The nutrients are broadly classified into two categories, namely, micronutrients and macronutrients. Some of the micronutrients are vitamins and minerals while carbohydrates, proteins and fats fall under macronutrients. The topics elaborated in this chapter will help in gaining a better perspective about these different types of essential nutrients.; **Chapter 4** - The purpose of food supplements is to provide nutrients which an individual is not able to obtain through normal diet, or is consuming in insufficient quantities. The diverse applications as well as the health benefits of food supplements have been thoroughly discussed in this chapter.; **Chapter 5** - A chemical substance which is added to food in order to produce particular desirable effects is known as a food additive. Anticaking agents, food coloring and sugar substitutes are a few examples of commonly used food additives. The diverse applications of these additives have been thoroughly discussed in this chapter.; **Chapter 6** - Food science and nutrition deal with a lot of processes which are associated with food such as food safety, food preservation and food fortification. It also includes sub-disciplines like food chemistry, food biotechnology and food microbiology. This chapter discusses in detail these processes and disciplines related to food science and nutrition.

Finally, I would like to thank my fellow scholars who gave constructive feedback and my family members who supported me at every step.

Theo Graham

Chapter 1

Food Science and Technology

The branch of science which deals with the study of the chemical, physical and biological makeup of food is known as food science. Food technology is involved in the study of the fundamental phenomena which are connected to the production of food products as well as their properties. This is an introductory chapter which will introduce briefly all the significant aspects of food science and technology.

Food Science

Food science is a discipline which studies chemical, biological, physical and other processes that have an influence on food's safety, flavour, appearance, etc. But it is also interested in other food-related practices and activities including design, packaging, new product development, optimisation of food manufacturing processes and similar.

The main goal of food science is to ensure that food products on store shelves are safe, tasty and nutritious. But in the recent years, food scientists have also started to pay more attention to informing and educating the public about the importance of proper food handling, storage and processing. The aim is to reduce the incidence of food-borne illnesses and help consumers prepare tasty meals that are packed with vitamins, minerals and other essential nutrients.

Food Microbiology

Basically the study of how microorganisms interact with foods, food microbiology focuses on bacteria, molds, yeasts and viruses. Areas of particular importance to product development are food safety and quality. Food safety deals with preventing pathogens in foods. It's nearly impossible to eliminate microorganisms from any food, but many steps can be taken to slow their growth or inactivate them. What food science is doing in the way of food safety is developing very sensitive and rapid techniques to identify pathogenic microorganisms and the toxins they produce in foods, and developing packaging and processes that inhibit their growth and reduce their rate of survival. Not all microorganisms are harmful, but some cause food spoilage.

The key to controlling spoilage is killing as many bacteria as we can without also killing the quality of the food in which they reside. Food microbiology is one of the most important fields of food science when it comes to product development, especially in this age of litigation. When devising a development plan for a new product, it is essential to consider the microbial quality of each component and how that may affect the overall quality of the product—and to determine how to process the product so that it has a sufficient shelf life.

Food Engineering and Processing

As far as product developers go, food engineers develop the concepts that processors use to turn raw ingredients into safe, long-lasting foods. In menu development, engineers may not play a direct role, but processors will. How an ingredient is processed can have a dramatic effect on the flavor, color, safety and shelf life of food. Consider high-pressure processing (HPP) and its effect on the fresh fruit and vegetable juice industry. HPP is a non-thermal or "cold pasteurization" process developed to allow fruit and vegetable juices to be produced without any of the deleterious effects of thermal treatments, such as changes in flavor, texture or color. The nutritional profile of the juices is unaltered by the process, so fortification is not necessary.

An all-natural, healthy and flavorful product can be produced thanks to food processing engineers. HPP can also be used to process raw clams, destroying potentially harmful bacteria. Think of the potential in a seafood restaurant chain. Clams, even oysters could be kept alive until the customer orders them; place the clams/oysters in the HPP and in a minute they're shucked and cleared of potentially harmful microorganisms.

Food Chemistry and Biochemistry

All foods are biochemicals because in most cases foods or their raw ingredients are or were living entities. Understanding biochemistry can be of vital importance to a product developer. Take the activity of enzymes. Adding the enzyme lactase to milk cuts the disaccharide lactose into its individual components galactose and glucose, making it more digestible. This opens up a whole spectrum of products for the lactose-intolerant. But the enzyme has an optimal activity at a specific pH and temperature—it won't survive certain types of processing. A grounding in biochemistry provides the knowledge to develop a product that takes advantage of such compounds.

Sensory Analysis

Sensory science uses people to describe and evaluate flavors, textures, appearance and other attributes of foods. Sensory evaluation practices are integral to product developers. Sensory techniques can be used to narrow down concepts and choose protocepts, optimize a developing product and monitor and control quality of the finished product. Consumer tests can be used to evaluate preference and acceptance of a product. Products can be evaluated and optimized using quantitative descriptive analysis (QDA), in which a focus group defines the sensory attributes for a product and establishes numerical scores for these attributes. Establishing the appropriate measurement is of major importance, as it allows sensory results to be quantified. This is the essence of sensory science: converting human perception of a food into quantifiable results.

Food Technology

Food Technology is a science which deals with the techniques and principles involved in processing and preserving the food substances. The application of food science helps in manufacturing safe, wholesome and nutritious food products. The study of food technology is to develop new methods and systems for keeping food products safe and resistant from natural harms such as bacteria and other micro-organisms. Food processing helps in preservation enhances the flavor and reduces the toxins in the food product which results in better distributional efficiency and easy marketing of the food product.

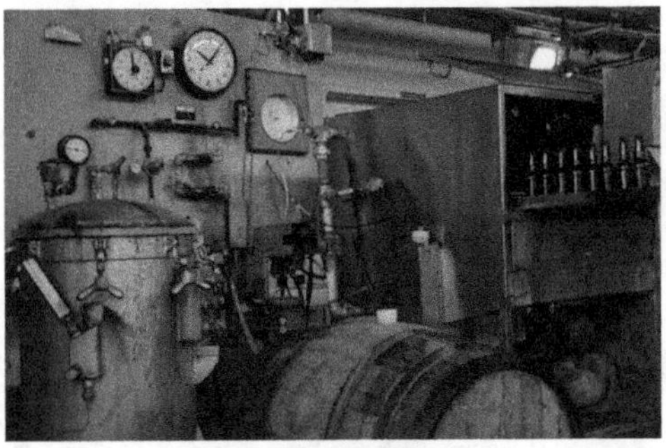

The modern food processing techniques is the key to flourishing supermarkets we have today. Extra nutrients can be added while processing the food and processed food is less susceptible to spoilage. Some of the techniques used are spray drying, juice concentrates, freeze drying and the introduction of artificial sweeteners, colorants, and preservatives. Of late, many products such as dried instant soups, reconstituted fruits and juices, and self-cooking meals were developed for the convenience of working people.

The food processing industries are involved in processes such as primary and secondary processing, preservation, quality management, packaging and labeling of a variety of products such as dairy products, fish products, fruit & vegetable products, meat & poultry products, confectionery products and food grains.

Few specializations in this field are:

- Dairy,
- Sugar,
- Alcohol,

- Bakery and confectionery items,
- Oil and oil seed processing,
- Fruits and vegetables,
- Meat- Fish,
- Cereals.

Food Processing

Food processing is the set of methods and techniques used to transform raw ingredients into food or food into other forms for consumption by humans or animals either in the home or by the food processing industry. Food processing typically takes clean, harvested crops or slaughtered and butchered animal products and uses these to produce attractive, marketable, and often long-life food products. Similar processes are used to produce animal feed. Extreme examples of food processing include the expert removal of toxic portions of the fugu fish or preparing space food for consumption under zero gravity.

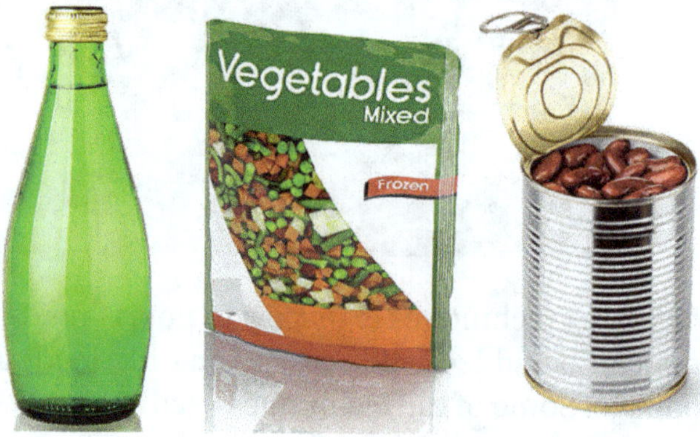

Examples of some processed foods

The benefits of food processing include the preservation, distribution, and marketing of food, protection from pathogenic microbes and toxic substances, year-round availability of many food items, and ease of preparation by the consumer. On the other hand, food processing can lower the nutritional value of foods, and processed foods may include additives (such as colorings, flavorings, and preservatives) that may have adverse health effects.

Food Processing Methods

Common food processing techniques include:

- Removal of unwanted outer layers, such as potato peeling or the skinning of peaches,

- Chopping or slicing, such as to produce diced carrots,
- Mincing and macerating,
- Liquefaction, such as to produce fruit juice,
- Fermentation, as in beer breweries,
- Emulsification,
- Cooking, by methods such as baking, boiling, broiling, frying, steaming, or grilling,
- Mixing,
- Addition of gas such as air entrainment for bread or gasification of soft drinks,
- Proofing,
- Spray drying,
- Pasteurization and
- Packaging.

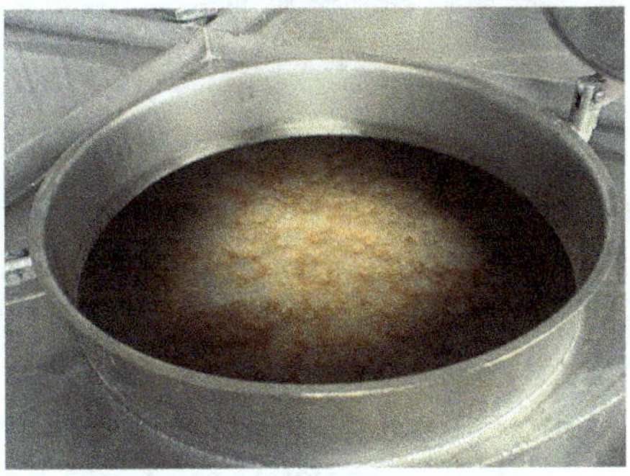

Beer fermenting at a brewery

Performance Parameters for Food Processing

When designing processes for the food industry, the following performance parameters may be taken into account:

- Hygiene, measured, for instance, by the number of microorganisms per ml of finished product.
- Energy consumption, measured, for instance, by "ton of steam per ton of sugar produced".
- Minimization of waste, measured, for instance, by the "percentage of peeling loss during the peeling of potatoes".

- Labor used, measured, for instance, by the "number of working hours per ton of finished product".
- Minimization of cleaning stops, measured, for instance, by the "number of hours between cleaning stops".

Benefits

More and more people live in the cities far away from where food is grown and produced. In many families, the adults are work from home and therefore there is little time for the preparation of food based on fresh ingredients. The food industry offers products that fulfill many different needs: from peeled potatoes that simply need to be boiled at home to fully prepared ready meals that can be heated up in the microwave oven in a few minutes.

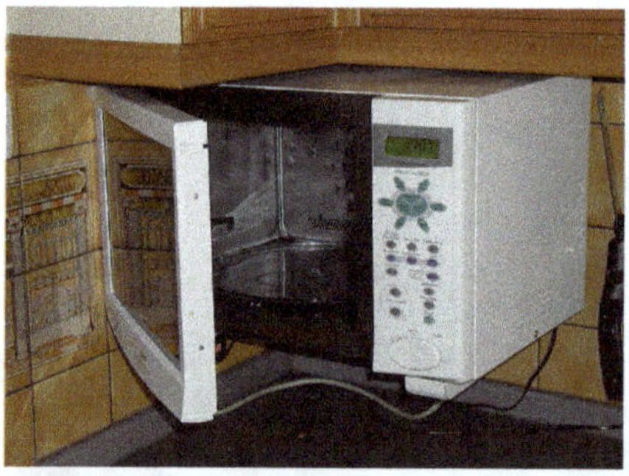

Microwave oven

Benefits of food processing include toxin removal, preservation, easing marketing and distribution tasks, and increasing food consistency. In addition, it increases seasonal availability of many foods, enables transportation of delicate perishable foods across long distances, and makes many kinds of foods safe to eat by de-activating spoilage and pathogenic micro-organisms. Modern supermarkets would not be feasible without modern food processing techniques, long voyages would not be possible, and military campaigns would be significantly more difficult and costly to execute.

Modern food processing also improves the quality of life for allergy sufferers, diabetics, and other people who cannot consume some common food elements. Food processing can also add extra nutrients such as vitamins.

Processed foods are often less susceptible to early spoilage than fresh foods, and are better suited for long distance transportation from the source to the consumer. Fresh materials, such as fresh produce and raw meats, are more likely to harbor pathogenic microorganisms (for example, Salmonella) capable of causing serious illnesses.

Drawbacks

In general, fresh food that has not been processed other than by washing and simple kitchen preparation, may be expected to contain a higher proportion of naturally occurring vitamins, fiber and minerals than the equivalent product processed by the food industry. Vitamin C, for example, is destroyed by heat and therefore canned fruits have a lower content of vitamin C than fresh ones.

Food processing can lower the nutritional value of foods. Processed foods tend to include food additives, such as flavorings and texture enhancing agents, which may have little or no nutritive value, and some may be unhealthy. Some preservatives added or created during processing, such as nitrites or sulfites, may cause adverse health effects.

Processed foods often have a higher ratio of calories to other essential nutrients than unprocessed foods, a phenomenon referred to as "empty calories." Most junk foods are processed, and fit this category.

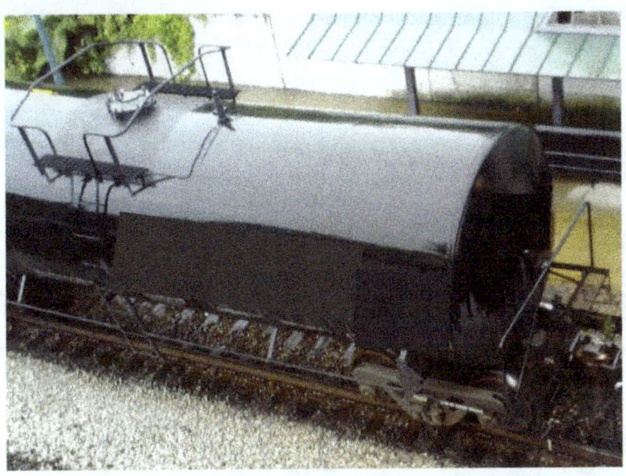

High quality and hygiene standards must be maintained to ensure consumer safety, and failure to maintain adequate standards can have serious health consequences.

Processing food is a very costly process, thus increasing the prices of foods products.

Trends in Modern Food Processing

Health

- Reduction of fat content in final product, for example, by using baking instead of deep-frying in the production of potato chips.
- Maintaining the natural taste of the product, for example, by using less artificial sweetener.

Hygiene

The rigorous application of industry and government endorsed standards to minimize possible risk and hazards. In the U.S., the standard adopted is HACCP.

Efficiency

- Rising energy costs lead to increasing usage of energy-saving technologies, for example, frequency converters on electrical drives, heat insulation of factory buildings, and heated vessels, energy recovery systems.
- Factory automation systems (often Distributed control systems) reduce personnel costs and may lead to more stable production results.

Industries

Food processing industries and practices include the following:

- Cannery,
- Industrial rendering,
- Meat packing plant,
- Slaughterhouse,
- Sugar industry,
- Vegetable packing plant.

References

- Fields-food-science: restaurantbusinessonline.com, Retrieved 2 March, 2019
- Food-Technology, Engineering-branches: myklassroom.com, Retrieved 12 August, 2019
- Food-processing: newworldencyclopedia.org, Retrieved 18 January, 2019
- Themes: esof2008.org, Retrieved 8 June, 2019

Chapter 2

Understanding Nutrition

The science of interpreting the interactions between nutrients and other materials in food with respect to the growth, health and disease in an organism is known as nutrition. Some of the sub-disciplines within nutrition are malnutrition and sports nutrition. The chapter closely examines these key concepts of nutrition to provide an extensive understanding of the subject.

Nutrition is defined as the processes by which an animal or plant takes in and utilises food substances. Essential nutrients include protein, carbohydrate, fat, vitamins, minerals and electrolytes. Normally, 85% of daily energy use is from fat and carbohydrates and 15% from protein. In humans, nutrition is mainly achieved through the process of putting foods into our mouths, chewing and swallowing it. The required amounts of the essential nutrients differ by age and the state of the body.

Nutrition is essential for growth and development, health and wellbeing. Eating a healthy diet contributes to preventing future illness and improving quality and length of life. Your nutritional status is the state of your health as determined by what you eat. There are several ways of assessing nutritional status, including anthropometric (i.e. physical body measurement), food intake and biochemical measurement.

Nutrients

Some precursors (i.e., the substances from which other substances are formed) of cell materials can be synthesized by the cell from other materials, while others must be supplied in foods. All the inorganic materials required for growth, together with an assortment of organic compounds whose number may vary from 1 to 30 or more, depending on the organism, fall into the latter category. Although organisms are able to synthesize nonessential nutrients, such nutrients are frequently utilized directly if present in food, thereby saving the organism the need to expend the energy required to synthesize them.

Inorganic Nutrients

A number of inorganic elements (minerals) are essential for the growth of living things. Boron, for example, has been demonstrated to be required for the growth of many—perhaps all—higher plants but has not been implicated as an essential element in the nutrition of either microorganisms or animals. Trace amounts of fluorine (as fluoride) are certainly beneficial, and perhaps essential, for proper tooth formation in higher animals. Similarly, iodine (as iodide) is required in animals for formation of thyroxine, the active component of an important regulatory hormone. Silicon (as silicate) is a prominent component of the outer skeletons of diatomaceous protozoans and similar organisms and is required in them for normal growth. In higher animals the requirement for silicon is much smaller. A less obvious example of a specialized mineral requirement is provided by calcium, which is required by higher animals in comparatively large amounts because it is a major component of bone and eggshells (in birds); for other organisms, calcium is an essential nutrient but only as a trace element. Mineral elements in wide variety are present in trace amounts in almost all foodstuffs. It cannot be assumed that the nonessential mineral elements play no useful role in metabolism.

Important antagonistic relationships between certain mineral nutrients also are known. A large excess of rubidium, for example, interferes with the utilization of potassium in some lactic-acid bacteria; zinc can interfere with manganese utilization in the same organism. In animal nutrition, excessive molybdenum or zinc (both of which are essential minerals) interferes with the utilization of copper, another essential mineral, and, in higher plants, excessive zinc can lead to a disorder that is known as iron chlorosis. Proper nutrient growth media for microorganisms and plants or diets for animals, therefore, require not only that the essential mineral elements be provided in sufficient amounts but also that they be used in the proper ratios to each other.

Organic Nutrients

The organic nutrients are the necessary building blocks of various cell components that certain organisms cannot synthesize and therefore must obtain preformed. These compounds include carbohydrates, protein, and lipids. Other organic nutrients include the vitamins, which are required in small amounts, because of either the catalytic role or the regulatory role they play in metabolism.

Interdependency of Nutritional Requirements

Competition for Sites of Absorption by the Cell

Since absorption of nutrients frequently occurs by way of active transport within cell membranes, an excess of one nutrient (A) may inhibit absorption of a second nutrient (B), if they share the same absorption pathway. In such cases, the apparent requirement for nutrient B increases; B, however, can sometimes be supplied in an alternate form that is able to enter the cell by a different route. Many examples of amino acid antagonism, in which inhibition of growth by one amino acid is counteracted by another amino acid, are best explained by this mechanism. For example, under some conditions Lactobacillus casei requires both D- and L-alanine, which differ from each other only in the position of the amino, or NH2, group in the molecule, and the two forms of this amino acid share the same absorption pathway. Excess D-alanine inhibits growth of this species, but the inhibition can be alleviated either by supplying additional L-alanine or, more effectively, by supplying peptides of L-alanine. The peptides enter the cell by a pathway different from that of the two forms of alanine and, after they are in the cell, can be broken down to form L-alanine. Relationships of this type provide one explanation for the fact that peptides are frequently more effective than amino acids in promoting growth of bacteria.

Competition for Sites of Utilization within the Cell

This phenomenon is similar to that regarding competition for absorption sites, but it occurs inside the cell and only between structurally similar nutrients (e.g., leucine and valine; serine and threonine).

Precursor-product Relationships

The requirement of rats and humans for the essential amino acids phenylalanine and methionine is substantially reduced if tyrosine, which is formed from phenylalanine, or cysteine, which is formed from methionine, is added to the diet. These relationships are explained by the fact that tyrosine and cysteine are synthesized in animals from phenylalanine and methionine, respectively. When the former (product) amino acids are supplied preformed, the latter (precursor) amino acids are required in smaller amounts. Several instances of the sparing of one nutrient by another because they have similar precursor-product relationships have been identified in other organisms.

Changes in Metabolic Pathways within the Cell

Rats fed diets containing large amounts of fat require substantially less thiamin (vitamin B1) than do those fed diets high in carbohydrate. The utilization of carbohydrate as an energy source (i.e., for ATP formation) is known to involve an important thiamin-dependent step, which is bypassed when fat is used as an energy source, and it is assumed that the lessened requirement for thiamin results from the change in metabolic pathways.

Syntrophism

Since the nutritional requirements and metabolic activities of organisms differ, it is clear that two or more different organisms growing relatedly may produce different overall changes in the environment. A rough example is provided by a balanced aquarium, in which aquatic plants utilize light and the waste products of animals—e.g., carbon dioxide, water, ammonia—to synthesize cell materials and generate oxygen, which in turn provide the materials necessary for animal growth. Such relationships are common among microorganisms; i.e., intermediate or end products of metabolism of one organism may provide essential nutrients for another. The mixed populations that result in nature provide examples of this phenomenon, which is called syntrophism; in some instances, the relationship may be so close as to constitute nutritional symbiosis, or mutualism. Several examples of this phenomenon have been found among thiamin-requiring yeasts and fungi, certain of which (group A) synthesized the thiazole component of thiamin molecule but require the pyrimidine portion preformed; for a second group (group B), the relationship is reversed. When group A and group B are grown together in a thiamin-free medium, both types of organisms survive, since each organism synthesizes the growth factor required by its partner; neither organism grows alone under these same conditions. Thus, two or more types of microorganisms frequently grow in situations in which only one species would not.

Such nutritional interrelationships may explain the fact that the nutritionally demanding lactic-acid bacteria are able to coexist with the nutritionally non-demanding coliform bacteria in the intestinal tracts of animals. It is known that the bacterial flora of the intestinal tract synthesize sufficient amounts of certain vitamins (e.g., vitamin K, folic acid) so that detection of deficiency symptoms in rats requires special measures, and the role of rumen bacteria in ruminant animals (e.g., cows, sheep) in rendering otherwise indigestible cellulose and other materials available to the host animal is well-known. These few examples indicate that syntrophic interrelationships are widespread in nature and may contribute substantially to the nutrition of a wide variety of species.

Nutritional Evolution of Organisms

Little is known about the nutritional evolution of living organisms. Nucleic acids, proteins, carbohydrates, and fats, which are present in all living cells, are formed by specific reaction sequences from a limited number of smaller compounds, most of which are common to all living organisms and, according to current theories, were available on Earth before life arose. Since less complex metabolic organization and less energy are required to synthesize cellular proteins from preformed amino acids than from carbon dioxide and other precursors, it is assumed that the simplest early forms of life were heterotrophic organisms requiring many organic nutrients for growth and that they selected such nutrients from their surroundings. As the supply of these preformed substances was exhausted, the organisms presumably developed the capacity to synthesize these preformed substances from simpler (precursor) materials present in the environment; in some organisms, this synthesizing capacity eventually evolved to the extent that carbon from carbon dioxide could be utilized to synthesize organic compounds.

At this point, autotrophy, as it now is known, became possible; autotrophy, in fact, may have evolved as a result of the exhaustion of the supply of preformed organic materials in the environment and the consequent necessity of organisms to synthesize the requirements themselves in order to survive. Implicit in this theory is the demonstrable assumption that autotrophic cells contain the most complex biosynthetic organization found in living things and that heterotrophic cells are simpler in that certain biosynthetic pathways do not occur. After the evolution of photosynthesis, a constantly renewable source of the organic compounds necessary for heterotrophic cell growth became available. It became feasible that those organisms whose environments provided a constantly available supply of a given compound could lose, through changes in their genetic material (mutations), the ability to synthesize that compound and still survive. Entire biosynthetic pathways may have been lost in this way; as long as such mutant organisms remained in an environment that supplied the necessary compound, the simplification in cellular organization and the energy saved by using preformed cell components would have given them a competitive advantage over the more complex parents from which they were derived and permitted stabilization of the mutation within the cell type. A theory that the requirements of modern organisms for essential organic nutrients arose through the loss of synthetic abilities present in more complex parent organisms was confirmed by the discovery that artificially produced mutant offspring of microorganisms can be readily obtained and may require the presence of one or more preformed organic compounds that the parent microorganisms could synthesize.

Human Nutrition

Human nutrition is the process by which substances in food are transformed into body tissues and provide energy for the full range of physical and mental activities that make up human life.

Utilization of Food by the Body

Calories and kilocalories: Energy Supply

The human body can be thought of as an engine that releases the energy present in the foods that it digests. This energy is utilized partly for the mechanical work performed by the muscles and in the secretory processes and partly for the work necessary to maintain the body's structure and functions. The performance of work is associated with the production of heat; heat loss is controlled so as to keep body temperature within a narrow range. Unlike other engines, however, the human body is continually breaking down (catabolizing) and building up (anabolizing) its component parts. Foods supply nutrients essential to the manufacture of the new material and provide energy needed for the chemical reactions involved.

Carbohydrate, fat, and protein are, to a large extent, interchangeable as sources of energy. Typically, the energy provided by food is measured in kilocalories, or Calories. One kilocalorie is equal to 1,000 gram-calories (or small calories), a measure of heat energy. However, in common parlance, kilocalories are referred to as "calories." In other words, a 2,000-calorie diet actually has 2,000 kilocalories of potential energy. One kilocalorie is the amount of heat energy required to raise one kilogram of water from 14.5 to 15.5 °C at one atmosphere of pressure. Another unit of energy widely used is the joule, which measures energy in terms of mechanical work. One joule is the energy expended when one kilogram is moved a distance of one metre by a force of one newton. The relatively higher levels of energy in human nutrition are more likely to be measured in kilojoules (1 kilojoule = 10^3 joules) or megajoules (1 megajoule = 10^6 joules). One kilocalorie is equivalent to 4.184 kilojoules.

The energy present in food can be determined directly by measuring the output of heat when the food is burned (oxidized) in a bomb calorimeter. However, the human body is not as efficient as a calorimeter, and some potential energy is lost during digestion and metabolism. Corrected physiological values for the heats of combustion of the three energy-yielding nutrients, rounded to whole numbers, are as follows: carbohydrate, 4 kilocalories (17 kilojoules) per gram; protein, 4 kilocalories (17 kilojoules) per gram; and fat, 9 kilocalories (38 kilojoules) per gram. Beverage alcohol (ethyl alcohol) also yields energy—7 kilocalories (29 kilojoules) per gram—although it is not essential in the diet. Vitamins, minerals, water, and other food constituents have no energy value, although many of them participate in energy-releasing processes in the body.

The energy provided by a well-digested food can be estimated if the gram amounts of energy-yielding substances (non-fibre carbohydrate, fat, protein, and alcohol) in that food are known. For example, a slice of white bread containing 12 grams of carbohydrate, 2 grams of protein, and 1 gram of fat supplies 67 kilocalories (280 kilojoules) of energy. Food composition tables and food labels provide useful data for evaluating energy and nutrient intake of an individual diet. Most foods provide a mixture of energy-supplying nutrients, along with vitamins, minerals, water, and other substances. Two notable exceptions are table sugar and vegetable oil, which are virtually pure carbohydrate (sucrose) and fat, respectively.

Throughout most of the world, protein supplies between 8 and 16 percent of the energy in the diet, although there are wide variations in the proportions of fat and carbohydrate in different populations. In more prosperous communities about 12 to 15 percent of energy is typically derived from protein, 30 to 40 percent from fat, and 50 to 60 percent from carbohydrate. On the other hand, in many poorer agricultural societies, where cereals comprise the bulk of the diet, carbohydrate provides an even larger percentage of energy, with protein and fat providing less. The human body is remarkably adaptable and can survive, and even thrive, on widely divergent diets. However, different dietary patterns are associated with particular health consequences.

BMR and REE: Energy Balance

Energy is needed not only when a person is physically active but even when the body is lying motionless. Depending on an individual's level of physical activity, between 50 and 80 percent of the energy expended each day is devoted to basic metabolic processes (basal metabolism), which enable the body to stay warm, breathe, pump blood, and conduct numerous physiological and biosynthetic activities, including synthesis of new tissue in growing children and in pregnant and lactating women. Digestion and subsequent processing of food by the body also uses energy and produces heat. This phenomenon, known as the thermic effect of food (or diet-induced thermogenesis), accounts for about 10 percent of daily energy expenditure, varying somewhat with the composition of the diet and prior dietary practices. Adaptive thermogenesis, another small but important component of energy expenditure, reflects alterations in metabolism due to changes in ambient temperature, hormone production, emotional stress, or other factors. Finally, the most variable component in energy expenditure is physical activity, which includes exercise and other voluntary activities as well as involuntary activities such as fidgeting, shivering, and maintaining posture. Physical activity accounts for 20 to 40 percent of the total energy expenditure, even less in a very sedentary person and more in someone who is extremely active.

Basal or resting energy expenditure is correlated primarily with lean body mass (fat-free mass and essential fat, excluding storage fat), which is the metabolically active tissue in the body. At rest, organs such as the liver, brain, heart, and kidney have the highest metabolic activity and, therefore, the highest need for energy, while muscle and bone require less energy, and body fat even less. Besides body composition, other factors affecting basal metabolism include age, sex, body temperature, and thyroid hormone levels.

The basal metabolic rate (BMR), a precisely defined measure of the energy expenditure necessary to support life, is determined under controlled and standardized conditions—shortly after awakening in the morning, at least 12 hours after the last meal, and with a comfortable room temperature. Because of practical considerations, the BMR is rarely measured; the resting energy expenditure (REE) is determined under less stringent conditions, with the individual resting comfortably about 2 to 4 hours after a meal. In practice, the BMR and REE differ by no more than 10 percent—the REE is usually slightly higher—and the terms are used interchangeably.

Energy expenditure can be assessed by direct calorimetry, or measurement of heat dissipated from the body, which employs apparatuses such as water-cooled garments or insulated chambers large enough to accommodate a person. However, energy expenditure is usually measured by the less cumbersome techniques of indirect calorimetry, in which heat produced by the body is calculated from measurements of oxygen inhaled, carbon dioxide exhaled, and urinary nitrogen excreted. The BMR (in kilocalories per day) can be roughly estimated using the following formula: $BMR = 70 \times (\text{body weight in kilograms})^{3/4}$.

The energy costs of various activities have been measured. While resting may require as little as 1 kilocalorie per minute, strenuous work may demand 10 times that much. Mental activity, though it may seem taxing, has no appreciable effect on energy requirement. A 70-kg (154-pound) man, whose REE over the course of a day might be 1,750 kilocalories, could expend a total of 2,400 kilocalories on a very sedentary day and up to 4,000 kilocalories on a very active day. A 55-kg (121-pound) woman, whose daily resting energy expenditure might be 1,350 kilocalories, could use from 1,850 to more than 3,000 total kilocalories, depending on level of activity.

The law of conservation of energy applies: If one takes in more energy than is expended, over time one will gain weight; insufficient energy intake results in weight loss, as the body taps its energy stores to provide for immediate needs. Excess food energy is stored in small amounts as glycogen, a short-term storage form of carbohydrate in muscle and liver, and as fat, the body's main energy reserve found in adipose tissue. Adipose tissue is mostly fat (about 87 percent), but it also contains some protein and water. In order to lose 454 grams (one pound) of adipose tissue, an energy deficit of about 3,500 kilocalories (14.6 megajoules) is required.

Body Mass, Body Fat and Body Water

The human body consists of materials similar to those found in foods; however, the relative proportions differ, according to genetic dictates as well as to the unique life experience of the individual. The body of a healthy lean man is composed of roughly 62 percent water, 16 percent fat, 16 percent protein, 6 percent minerals, and less than 1 percent carbohydrate, along with very small amounts of vitamins and other miscellaneous substances. Females usually carry more fat (about 22 percent in a healthy lean woman) and slightly less of the other components than do males of comparable weight.

The body's different compartments—lean body mass, body fat, and body water—are constantly adjusting to changes in the internal and external environment so that a state of dynamic equilibrium (homeostasis) is maintained. Tissues in the body are continuously being broken down (catabolism) and built up (anabolism) at varying rates. For example, the epithelial cells lining the digestive tract are replaced at a dizzying speed of every three or four days, while the life span of red blood cells is 120 days, and connective tissue is renewed over the course of several years.

Although estimates of the percentage of body fat can be made by direct inspection, this approach is imprecise. Body fat can be measured indirectly using fairly precise but costly methods, such as underwater weighing, total body potassium counting, and dual-energy X-ray absorptiometry (DXA). However, more practical, albeit less accurate, methods are often used, such as anthropometry, in which subcutaneous fat at various sites is measured using skinfold calipers; bioelectrical impedance, in which resistance to a low-intensity electrical current is used to estimate body fat; and near infrared interactance, in which an infrared light aimed at the biceps is used to assess fat and protein interaction. Direct measurement of the body's various compartments can only be performed on cadavers.

The composition of the body tends to change in somewhat predictable ways over the course of a lifetime—during the growing years, in pregnancy and lactation, and as one ages—with corresponding changes in nutrient needs during different phases of the life cycle. Regular physical exercise can help attenuate the age-related loss of lean tissue and increase in body fat.

Food Groups

The following nine food groups reflect foods with generally similar nutritional characteristics:

(1) Cereals,

(2) Starchy roots,

(3) Legumes,

(4) Vegetables and fruits,

(5) Sugars, preserves, and syrups,

(6) Meat, fish, and eggs,

(7) Milk and milk products,

(8) Fats and oils,

(9) Beverages.

Cereals

The cereals are all grasses that have been bred over millennia to bear large seeds (i.e., grain). The most important cereals for human consumption are rice, wheat, and corn (maize). Others include barley, oats, and millet. The carbohydrate-rich cereals compare favourably with the protein-rich foods in energy value; in addition, the cost of production (per calorie) of cereals is less than that of almost all other foods and they can be stored dry for many years. Therefore, most of the world's diets are arranged to meet main calorie requirements from the cheaper carbohydrate foods. The major component of all grains is starch. Cereals contain little fat, with oats having an exceptional 9 percent. The amount of protein in cereals ranges from 6 to 16 percent but does not have as high a nutritive value as that of many animal foods because of the low lysine content.

Controversy exists as to the relative merits of white bread and bread made from whole wheat flour. White flour consists of about 72 percent of the grain but contains little of the germ (embryo) and of the outer coverings (bran). Since the B vitamins are concentrated mainly in the scutellum (covering of the germ), and to a lesser extent in the bran, the vitamin B content of white flour, unless artificially enriched, is less than that of brown flour. Dietary fibre is located mostly in the bran, so that white flour contains only about one-third of that in whole wheat flour. White flour is compulsorily enriched with synthetic vitamins in a number of countries, including the United States and the United Kingdom, so that the vitamin content is similar to that of the darker flours. White flour still lacks fibre and any yet unidentified beneficial factors that may be present in the outer layers of the wheat.

B vitamins are also lost when brown rice is polished to yield white rice. People living on white rice and little else are at risk for developing the disease beriberi, which is caused by a deficiency of thiamin (vitamin B1). Beriberi was formerly common in poor Asian communities in which a large proportion of the diet consisted of polished rice. The disease has almost completely disappeared from Asia with the advent of greater availability of other foods and, in some areas, fortification of the rice with thiamin.

Yellow corn differs from other cereals in that it contains carotenoids with vitamin A activity. (Another exception is a genetically modified so-called golden rice, which contains carotene, the precursor for vitamin A.) Corn is also lower in the amino acid tryptophan than other cereals. The niacin in corn is in a bound form that cannot be digested or absorbed by humans unless pretreated with lime (calcium hydroxide) or unless immature grains are eaten at the so-called milky stage (usually as sweet corn). Niacin is also formed in the body as a metabolite of the amino acid tryptophan, but this alternative source is not available when the tryptophan content is too low.

Starchy Roots

Starchy roots consumed in large quantities include potatoes, sweet potatoes, yams, taro, and cassava. Their nutritive value in general resembles that of cereals. The potato, however, provides some protein (2 percent) and also contains vitamin C. The yellow-fleshed varieties of sweet potato contain the pigment beta-carotene, convertible in the body into vitamin A. Cassava is extremely low in protein, and most varieties contain cyanide-forming compounds that make them toxic unless processed correctly.

Legumes

Beans and peas are the seeds of leguminous crops that are able to utilize atmospheric nitrogen via parasitic microorganisms attached to their roots. Legumes contain at least 20 percent protein, and they are a good source of most of the B vitamins and of iron. Like cereals, most legumes are low in fat; an important exception is the soybean (17 percent), a major commercial source of edible oil.

Vegetables and Fruits

Vegetables and fruits have similar nutritive properties. Because 70 percent or more of their weight is water, they provide comparatively little energy or protein, but many contain vitamin C and carotene. However, cooked vegetables are an uncertain source of vitamin C, as this vitamin is easily destroyed by heat. The dark-green leafy vegetables are particularly good sources of vitamin A activity. Vegetables also provide calcium and iron but often in a form that is poorly absorbed. The more typical fruits, such as apples, oranges, and berries, are rich in sugar. Bananas are a good source of potassium. Vegetables and fruits also contain fibre, which adds bulk to the intestinal content and is useful in preventing constipation.

Botanically, nuts are actually a kind of fruit, but they are quite different in character with their hard shell and high fat content. The coconut, for example, contains some 60 percent fat when dried. Olives are another fruit rich in fat and are traditionally grown for their oil.

Sugars, Preserves and Syrups

One characteristic of diets of affluent societies is their high content of sugar. This is due in part to sugar added at the table or as an ingredient in candy, preserves, and sweetened colas or other beverages. There are also naturally occurring sugars in foods (lactose in milk and fructose, glucose, and sucrose in fruits and some vegetables). Sugar, however, contains no protein, minerals, or vitamins and thus has been called the source of "empty calories."

Because sugar adsorbs water and prevents the growth of microorganisms, it is an excellent preservative. Making jam or marmalade is a way of preserving fruit, but most of the vitamin C is destroyed, and the products contain up to 70 percent sugar. Honey and natural syrups (e.g., maple syrup) are composed of more than 75 percent sugar.

Meat, Fish and Eggs

Generally meats consist of about 20 percent protein, 20 percent fat, and 60 percent water. The amount of fat present in a particular portion of meat varies greatly, not only with the kind of meat but also with the quality; the "energy value" varies in direct proportion with the fat content. Meat is valuable for its protein, which is of high biological value. Pork is an excellent source of thiamin. Meat is also a good source of niacin, vitamin B_{12}, vitamin B_6, and the mineral nutrients iron, zinc, phosphorus, potassium, and magnesium. Liver is the storage organ for, and is very rich in, vitamin A, riboflavin, and folic acid. In many cultures the organs (offal) of animals—including the kidneys, the heart, the tongue, and the liver—are considered delicacies. Liver is a particularly rich source of many vitamins.

The muscular tissue of fishes consists of 13 to 20 percent protein, fat ranging from less than 1 to more than 20 percent, and 60 to 82 percent water that varies inversely with fat content. Many species of fish, such as cod and haddock, concentrate fat in the liver and as a result have extremely lean muscles. The tissues of other fish, such as salmon and herring, may contain 15 percent fat or more. However, fish oil, unlike the fat in land animals, is rich in essential long-chain fatty acids, particularly eicosapentaenoic acid.

The egg has a deservedly high reputation as a food. Its white contains protein, and its yolk is rich in both protein and vitamin A. An egg also provides calcium and iron. Egg yolk, however, has a high cholesterol content.

Milk and Milk Products

The milk of each species of animal is a complete food for its young. Moreover, one pint of cow's milk contributes about 90 percent of the calcium, 30 to 40 percent of the riboflavin, 25 to 30 percent of the protein, 10 to 20 percent of the calories and vitamins A and B, and up to 10 percent of the iron and vitamin D needed by a human adult.

Human breast milk is the perfect food for infants, provided it comes from a healthy, well-nourished mother and the infant is full-term. Breast milk contains important antibodies, white blood cells, and nutrients. In communities where hygiene is poor, breast-fed babies have fewer infections than formula-fed babies. In the past, infants who could not be breast-fed were given cow's milk that was partially "humanized" with the addition of water and a small amount of sugar or wheat flour. However, this was far from an ideal substitute for breast milk, being lower in iron and containing undenatured proteins that could produce allergic reactions with bleeding into the gut and, in some cases, eczema.

Lactose, the characteristic sugar of milk, is a disaccharide made of the monosaccharides glucose and galactose. Some adults can break down the lactose of large quantities of milk into galactose and glucose, but others have an inherited lactose intolerance as a result of the lactase enzyme no longer being secreted into the gut after the age of weaning. As a result, unabsorbed lactose is fermented by bacteria and produces bloating and gas. People who have little lactase in their bodies can still consume large amounts of milk if it has been allowed to go sour, if lactobacilli have split most of the lactose into lactic acid (as in yogurt), or if the lactose has been treated with commercially available lactase. People originating in northern Europe usually retain full intestinal lactase activity into adult life.

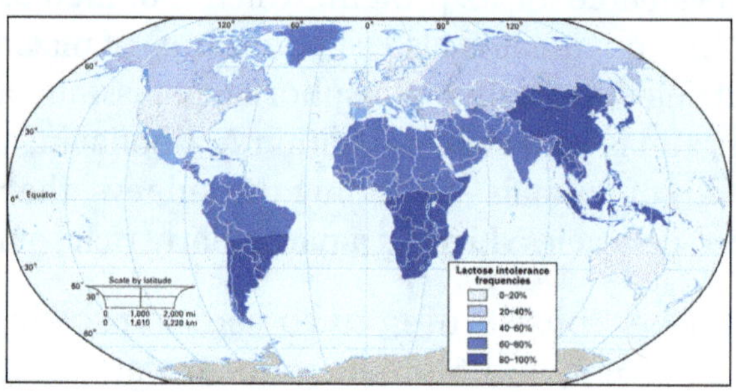

Lactose intolerance, global distribution: Global distribution of lactose intolerance in humans

Most commercially available milk has been pasteurized with heat to kill bovine tuberculosis organisms and other possible pathogens. The most widely used method for pasteurizing milk is the high-temperature, short-time (HTST) sterilization treatment. If products are to be stored under refrigeration, or even at room temperature, for long periods of time, they may be processed by ultrahigh temperature (UHT) pasteurization. Another method of preserving milk without refrigeration involves the removal of water to form condensed milk, which can be exposed to air for several days without deterioration. Milk, either whole or defatted, can also be dried to a powder. In some countries, such as the United States, milk is homogenized so that fat particles are broken up and evenly distributed throughout the product.

Cow's milk is good food for human adults, but the cream (i.e., the fat) contains 52 percent saturated fatty acids as compared with only 3 percent polyunsaturated fat. This fat is either drunk with the milk or eaten in butter or cream. Because milk fat is regarded as undesirable by people who want to reduce their energy intake or cholesterol level, the dairy industry has developed low-fat cow's milk (with 2 percent fat instead of the almost 4 percent of whole milk), very low-fat skim milk, and skim milk with extra nonfat milk solids (lactose, protein, and calcium) that give more body to the milk. Buttermilk, originally the watery residue of butter making, is now made from either low-fat or skim milk that has been inoculated with nonpathogenic bacteria.

Cheese making is an ancient art formerly used on farms to convert surplus milk into a food that could be stored without refrigeration. Rennet, an enzyme found in a calf's stomach, is added to milk, causing the milk protein casein to coagulate into a semisolid substance called curd, thus trapping most of the fat. The remaining watery liquid (whey) is then drained, and the curd is salted, inoculated with nonpathogenic organisms, and allowed to dry and mature. Cheese is rich in protein and calcium and is a good source of vitamin A and riboflavin. Most cheeses, however, contain about 25 to 30 percent fat (constituting about 70 percent of the calories of the cheese), which is mostly saturated, and they are usually high in sodium.

Fats and Oils

The animal fats used by humans are butter, suet (beef fat), lard (pork fat), and fish oils. Important vegetable oils include olive oil, peanut (groundnut) oil, coconut oil, cottonseed oil, sunflower seed oil, soybean oil, safflower oil, rape oil, sesame (gingelly) oil, mustard oil, red palm oil, and corn oil. Fats and oils provide more calories per gram than any other food, but they contain no protein and few micronutrients. Only butter and the previously mentioned fish-liver oils contain any vitamin A or D, though red palm oil does contain carotene, which is converted to vitamin A in the body. Vitamins A and D are added to margarines. All natural fats and oils contain variable amounts of vitamin E, the fat-soluble vitamin antioxidant.

The predominant substances in fats and oils are triglycerides, chemical compounds containing any three fatty acids combined with a molecule of glycerol. When no double bonds are present, a fatty acid is said to be saturated; with the presence of one or more double bonds, a fatty acid is said to be unsaturated. Fats with a high percentage of saturated fatty acids, e.g., butter and lard, tend to be solid at room temperature. Those with a high percentage of unsaturated fatty acids are usually liquid oils, e.g., sunflower, safflower, and corn oils. The process of hydrogenation is used by the food industry to convert unsaturated oils to saturated solid fats, which are more resistant to rancidity. However, hydrogenation also causes the formation of trans-fatty acids. These appear to have some of the same undesirable effects on blood cholesterol as saturated fatty acids.

A small group of fatty acids is essential in the diet. They occur in body structures, especially the different membranes inside and around cells, and cannot be synthesized in the body from other fats. Linoleic acid is the most important of these fatty acids because it is convertible to other essential fatty acids. Linoleic acid has two double bonds and is a polyunsaturated fatty acid. As well as being an essential fatty acid, it tends to lower the cholesterol level in the blood. Linoleic acid occurs in moderate to high proportions in many of the seed oils, e.g., corn, sunflower, cottonseed, and safflower oils. Some margarines (polyunsaturated margarines) use a blend of oils selected to provide a moderately high linoleic acid content.

Beverages

Although most adults drink one to two litres (about one to two quarts) of water a day, much of this is in the form of liquids such as coffee, tea, fruit juices, and soft drinks. In general, these are appreciated more for their taste or for their effects than for their nutritive value. Fruit juices are useful for their vitamin C content and are good sources of potassium; however, they tend to be very high in sugar. Coffee and tea by themselves are of little nutritive value; coffee contains some niacin, and tea contains fluoride and manganese. These beverages also contain natural caffeine, which has a stimulating effect. Caffeine is added to colas, and so-called diet soft drinks contain small quantities of artificial sweeteners in place of sugars so that their overall calorie value is reduced.

Since ethyl alcohol (ethanol) has an energy value of 7 kilocalories per gram, very significant amounts of energy can be obtained from alcoholic drinks. Beer contains 2 to 6 percent alcohol, wines 10 to 13 percent, and most spirits up to 40 percent. Fermented drinks also include significant amounts of residual sugars, and champagne and dessert wines may have sugar added to them. With one or two exceptions, alcoholic beverages contain no nutrients and are only a source of "empty calories." The only vitamin present in significant amounts in beer is riboflavin. Wines are devoid of vitamins but sometimes contain large amounts of iron, probably acquired from iron vessels used in their preparation. Heavy alcohol consumption is known to lead to a greater risk of malnutrition, in part because it can damage the absorptive power of the gut and also because heavy drinkers commonly neglect to follow a normal pattern of meals. On the other hand, evidence from a number of studies shows that persons consuming one to two drinks per day are healthier than are those who abstain from drinking alcohol. This might be due in part to substances in red wine, such as flavonoids and tannins, which may protect against heart disease.

Nutrition throughout the Life Cycle

Nutritional needs and concerns vary during different stages of life. Selected issues are discussed below:

Pregnancy and Lactation

A woman's nutritional status before and during pregnancy affects not only her own health but also the health and development of her baby. If a woman is underweight before becoming pregnant or fails to gain sufficient weight during pregnancy, her chance of having a premature or low-birth-weight infant is increased. Overweight women, on the other hand, have a high risk of complications during pregnancy, such as high blood pressure (hypertension) and gestational diabetes, and of having a poorly developed infant or one with birth defects. Weight loss during pregnancy is never recommended. Recommended weight gain during pregnancy is 11.5 to 16 kg (25 to 35 pounds) for a woman of normal weight—slightly more for an underweight woman and slightly less for an overweight woman.

Overall nutritional requirements increase with pregnancy. In the second and third trimesters, pregnant women need additional food energy—about 300 kilocalories above non-pregnant needs. Most additional nutrient needs can be met by selecting food wisely, but an iron supplement (30 milligrams per day) is usually recommended during the second and third trimesters, in addition to a folic acid supplement throughout pregnancy. Other key nutrients of particular concern are protein, vitamin D, calcium, and zinc.

Heavy alcohol consumption or "binge drinking" during pregnancy can cause fetal alcohol syndrome, a condition with irreversible mental and physical retardation. Even lighter social drinking during pregnancy may result in milder damage—growth retardation, behavioral or learning abnormalities, or motor impairments—sometimes described as fetal alcohol effects. Until a completely safe level of intake can be determined, pregnant women are advised not to drink at all, especially during the first trimester. Caffeine consumption is usually limited as a precautionary measure, and cigarette smoking is not advised under any circumstances. Limiting intake of certain fish, such as swordfish and shark, which may be contaminated with methylmercury, is also recommended.

An extra 500 kilocalories of food per day is needed to meet the energy demands of lactation. Because pregnancy depletes maternal iron stores, iron supplementation during lactation may be advised. Breast-fed infants may be sensitive to the constituents and flavours of foods and beverages consumed by the mother. In general, lactating women are advised to consume little, if any, alcohol.

Infancy, Childhood and Adolescence

Breast-fed infants, in general, have fewer infections and a reduced chance of developing allergies and food intolerances. For these and other reasons, breast-feeding is strongly recommended for at least the first four to six months of life. However, if a woman is unable to breast-feed or chooses not to, infant formulas (altered forms of cow's milk) can provide safe and adequate nourishment for an infant. Goat's milk, evaporated milk, and sweetened condensed milk are inappropriate for infants. Soy formulas and hydrolyzed protein formulas can be used if a milk allergy is suspected. In developing countries with poor sanitation, over-diluted formulas or those prepared with contaminated water can cause malnutrition and infection, resulting in diarrhea, dehydration, and even death. Breast-fed infants may need supplements of iron and vitamin D during the first six months of life and fluoride after six months. A vitamin B_{12} supplement is advised for breast-fed infants whose mothers are strict vegetarians (vegans).

Solid foods, starting with iron-fortified infant cereals, can be introduced between four and six months to meet nutrient needs that breast milk or infant formulas can no longer supply alone. Other foods can be introduced gradually, one every few days. Infants should not be given honey (which may contain bacteria that can cause botulism), foods that are too salty or sweet, foods that may cause choking, or large amounts of fruit juice.

Starting at one year of age, whole cow's milk can be an excellent source of nutrients for children. However, because cow's milk is associated with gastrointestinal blood loss, iron deficiency, and an allergic response in some young infants, some medical societies do not recommend giving unmodified whole cow's milk to children less than one year old. Low-fat or nonfat milk is inappropriate for children less than two years of age.

The rapid growth rate of infancy slows down in early childhood. During childhood—but not before the age of two—a gradual transition to lower-fat foods is recommended, along with regular exercise. Establishing healthful practices in childhood will reduce the risk of childhood obesity as well as obesity in adulthood and related chronic diseases (e.g., heart disease, diabetes, and high blood pressure).

Vegetarian children can be well nourished but care is needed for them to receive sufficient energy (calories), good-quality protein, vitamins B_{12} and D, and the minerals iron, zinc, and calcium. It is difficult for children who do not drink milk to obtain enough calcium from their food, and supplements may be required. Because of possible toxicity, iron supplements should be taken only under medical supervision.

A small percentage of school-age children who have difficulty sitting still and paying attention are diagnosed with attention-deficit/ hyperactivity disorder (ADHD). Studies have found no convincing evidence that ADHD is caused by sugar or food additives in the diet or that symptoms can be alleviated by eliminating these substances.

Because of unusual eating practices, skipped meals, and concerns about body image, many teenagers, especially girls, have a less than optimal diet. Teenage girls, in particular, need to take special care to obtain adequate amounts of calcium so that bones can be properly mineralized. Iron-deficiency anemia is a concern not only for teenage girls, who lose iron periodically in menstrual blood, but also for teenage boys.

Adulthood

No matter which nutritional and health practices are followed, the body continues to age, and there appears to be a strong genetic component to life expectancy. Nevertheless, healthful dietary practices and habits such as limited alcohol use, avoidance of tobacco products, and regular physical activity can help reduce the chance of premature death and increase the chance of vitality in the older years. For the most part, a diet that is beneficial for adults in general is also beneficial for people as they age, taking into account possible changes in energy needs.

In elderly people, common problems that contribute to inadequate nutrition are tooth loss, decreased sense of taste and smell, and a sense of isolation—all of which result in decreased food intake and weight loss. The elderly may have gastrointestinal ailments, such as poor absorption of vitamin B_{12}, and digestion difficulties, such as constipation. Inadequate fluid intake may lead to dehydration. Nutritional deficiency may further compromise declining immune function. Prescription and over-the-counter drugs may interact with nutrients and exacerbate the nutritional deficits of the elderly. In addition, decreasing physical activity, loss of muscle tissue, and increasing body fat are associated with type 2 diabetes, hypertension, and risk of cardiovascular disease and other diseases. Older people, especially those with reduced sun exposure or low intakes of fatty fish or vitamin D-fortified food, may need supplemental vitamin D to help preserve bone mass. Adequate calcium intake and weight-bearing exercise are also important, but these measures cannot completely stop the decline in bone density with age that makes both men and women vulnerable to bone fractures (due to osteoporosis), which could leave them bedridden and could even be life-threatening. Treatment with various bone-conserving drugs has been found to be effective in slowing bone loss. Staying physically fit as one ages can improve strength and balance, thereby preventing falls, contributing to overall health, and reducing the impact of aging.

There is evidence that intake of the antioxidants vitamin C, vitamin E, and beta-carotene as well as the mineral zinc may slow the progression of age-related macular degeneration, a leading cause of blindness in people older than 65 years. Two carotenoids, lutein and zeaxanthin, also are being studied for their possible role in protecting against age-related vision loss. Research suggests that the dietary supplement glucosamine, a substance that occurs naturally in the body and contributes to cartilage formation, may be useful in lessening the pain and disability of osteoarthritis. Aerobic exercise and strength training, as well as losing excess weight, also may provide some relief from arthritis pain.

Elevated blood levels of the amino acid homocysteine have been associated with an increased risk of cardiovascular disease and with Alzheimer disease, the most common form of dementia; certain B vitamins, particularly folic acid, may be effective in lowering homocysteine levels. High concentrations of aluminum in the brains of persons with Alzheimer disease are most likely a result of the disease and not a cause, as correspondingly high levels of aluminum are not found in blood and hair. There is ongoing research into the possible value of dietary supplements for the normal memory problems that beset healthy older people.

Eating a healthful diet, obtaining sufficient sleep, avoiding smoking, keeping physically fit, and maintaining an active mind are among the practices that may increase not only life expectancy but also the chance of a full and productive life in one's later years. The so-called free-radical theory of aging—the notion that aging is accelerated by highly reactive substances that damage cellular components, and that intake of various antioxidants can repair free-radical damage and thereby slow aging—has generated much interest and is a promising area of research, but it has not been scientifically established. On the contrary, the life spans of various mammalian species have not been extended significantly by antioxidant therapy. Ongoing studies are investigating whether the consumption of 30 percent fewer calories (undernutrition, not malnutrition) slows aging and age-related disease and extends life spans in nonhuman primates. There is no evidence that severe energy restriction would extend the human life span beyond its current maximum of 115 to 120 years.

Sports Nutrition

Sports nutrition is the foundation of athletic success. It is a well-designed nutrition plan that allows active adults and athletes to perform at their best. It supplies the right food type, energy, nutrients, and fluids to keep the body well hydrated and functioning at peak levels. A sports nutrition diet may vary day to day, depending on specific energy demands.

Sports Nutrition basics

Macronutrients

The energy required for living and physical activity comes from the food we eat and fluid intake. Macronutrients in the following food groups supply the energy essential to optimal body function:

- Carbohydrates are either simple or complex, and the most important energy source for the human body. Simple carbs include sugars naturally occurring in foods like fruits, vegetables, and milk. Whole grain bread, potatoes, most vegetables, and oats are examples of healthy complex carbs. Your digestive system breaks down carbohydrates into glucose or blood sugar which feeds energy to your cells, tissues, and organs.

- Proteins are made up of a chain of amino acids and are essential to every cell of the human body. Protein can either be complete or incomplete. A complete protein contains all the amino acids needed by the body, and include animal sources like meat, fish, poultry, and milk. Incomplete protein sources (typically plant-based proteins) often lack one or more of the essential amino acids. Essential amino acids can't be made by the body and must be supplied by food. Protein plays an important role in muscle recovery and growth.

- Fats can be saturated or unsaturated, and they play a vital role in the human body. Unsaturated fats are considered healthy and come from plant sources like olive oil and nuts. Saturated fats are found in animal products like red meats and high-fat dairy, which are indicated to increase the risk of disease. Healthy fats provide energy, help with body development, protect our organs, and maintain cell membranes.

The Goal of Sports Nutrition

Active adults and competitive athletes turn to sports nutrition to help them achieve their goals. Examples of individual goals could include gaining lean mass, improving body composition, or enhancing athletic performance. These sport-specific scenarios require differing nutritional programs. Research findings indicate the right food type, caloric intake, nutrient timing, fluids, and supplementation are essential and specific to each individual. The following are different states of training and competitive sport benefiting from sports nutrition:

Eating for Exercise/Athletic Performance

Training programs require a well-designed diet for active adults and competitive athletes. Research shows a balanced nutrition plan should include sufficient calories and healthy macronutrients to optimize athletic performance. The body will use carbohydrates or fats as the main energy source, depending on exercise intensity and duration. Inadequate caloric intake can impede athletic training and performance.

For example, and according to research, energy expenditure for extreme cyclists competing in the Tour de France is approximately 12,000 calories per day.

- Carbohydrates are the main fuel source for an active adult or competitive athlete. General guidelines for carbohydrate intake are based on body size and training characteristics. Carbohydrate needs in a daily diet can range from 45 to 65 percent of total food intake depending on physical demands.

- Proteins are responsible for muscle growth and recovery in the active adult or athlete. Sufficient amounts of protein per individual help maintain a positive nitrogen balance in the body, which is vital to muscle tissue. Protein requirements can vary significantly ranging from 0.8g to 2g per kilogram of body weight per day.

- Fats help maintain energy balance, regulate hormones, and restore muscle tissue. Omega-3 and omega-6 are essential fatty acids that are especially important to a sports nutrition diet. Research findings recommend an athlete consume approximately 30 percent of their total daily caloric intake as a healthy fat.

Eating for Endurance

Endurance programs are defined as one to three hours per day of moderate to high-intensity exercise. High-energy intake in the form of carbohydrates is essential. According to research, target carbohydrate consumption for endurance athletes ranges from 6g to 10g per kilogram of body weight per day. Fat is a secondary source of energy used during long-duration training sessions. Endurance athletes are more at risk for dehydration. Replacing fluids and electrolytes lost through sweat are necessary for peak performance.

Eating for Strength

Resistance training programs are designed to gradually build the strength of skeletal muscle. Strength training is high-intensity work. It requires sufficient amounts of all macronutrients for muscle development. Protein intake is especially vital to increase and maintain lean body mass. Research indicates protein requirements can vary from 1.2g to 3.1g per kilogram of body weight per day.

Eating for Competition

Preparing for a competitive sport will vary in sports nutrition requirements. For example, strength athletes strive to increase lean mass and body size for their sport. Endurance runners focus on reduced body weight/fat for peak body function during their event. Athletic goals will determine the best sports nutrition strategy. Pre and post-workout meal planning are unique for each athlete and essential for optimal performance.

Hydration and Sports Performance

Adequate hydration and electrolytes are essential for health and athletic performance. We all lose water throughout the day, but active adults and athletes lose additional body water (and a significant amount of sodium) sweating during intense workouts.

Dehydration is the process of losing body water, and fluid deficits greater than 2 percent of body weight can compromise athletic performance and cognitive function. Athletes are recommended to use fluid replacement strategies as part of their sports nutrition to maintain optimal body functioning. Rehydration with water and sports drinks containing sodium are often consumed depending on the athlete and sporting event. Lack of sufficient hydration for athletes may lead to the following:

- Hypohydration (dehydration).
- Hypovolemia (decreased plasma/blood volume).
- Hyponatremia (low blood sodium levels/water intoxication).

Supplements in Sports Nutrition

Sports supplements and foods are unregulated products marketed to enhance athletic performance. According to the Academy of Sports Medicine, “the ethical use of sports supplements is a personal choice and remains controversial." There are limited supplements backed by clinical research. The Institute of Sport has provided a general guide ranking sports performance supplements and foods according to the significance of scientific evidence:

- Sports food: sports drinks, bars, and gels, electrolyte supplements, protein supplements, liquid meal supplements.
- Medical supplements: iron, calcium, vitamin D, multi-vitamin/mineral, omega-3 fatty acids.
- Performance supplements: creatine, caffeine, sodium bicarbonate, beta-alanine, nitrate.

Sports Nutrition for Special Populations and Environments

Sports nutrition covers a wide spectrum of needs for athletes. Certain populations and environments require additional guidelines and information to enhance athletic performance.

- Vegetarian athlete: A vegetarian diet contains high intakes of plant proteins, fruits, vegetables, whole grains, and nuts. It can be nutritionally adequate, but insufficient evidence exists on long-term vegetarianism and athletic performance. Dietary assessments are recommended to avoid deficiencies and to ensure adequate nutrients to support athletic demands.
- High altitude: Specialized training and nutrition are required for athletes training at high altitude. Increasing red blood cells to carry more oxygen is essential. Iron-rich foods are an important component for this athlete as well. Increased risk of illness is indicated with chronic high altitude exposure. Foods high in antioxidants and protein are essential. Fluid requirements will vary per athlete, and hydration status should be individually monitored.
- Hot environments: Athletes competing in hot conditions are at greater risk of heat illness. Heat illness can have adverse health complications. Fluid and electrolyte balance is crucial for these athletes. Hydration strategies are required to maintain peak performance while exercising in the heat.
- Cold environments: Primary concerns for athletes exercising in the cold are adequate hydration and body temperature. Leaner athletes are at higher risk of hypothermia. Modifying caloric and carbohydrate intake are important for this athlete. Appropriate foods and fluids that withstand cold temperatures will promote optimal athletic performance.

Special Topics in Sports Nutrition

Eating disorders in athletes are not uncommon. Many athletes are required to maintain lean bodies and low body weight and exhibit muscular development. Chronic competitive pressure can create psychological and physical stress of the athlete leading to disordered eating habits. Without proper counseling, adverse health effects may eventually develop. The most common eating disorders among athletes may include:

- Anorexia nervosa,
- Bulimia,
- Compulsive exercise disorder,
- Orthorexia.

Obviously, the nutritional needs of these individuals greatly differ from that of other active adults or athletes. Until someone with an eating disorder is considered well again, the primary focus should be put on treating and managing the eating disorder and consuming the nutrition needed to achieve and maintain good health, rather than athletic performance.

Micronutrient deficiencies are a concern for active adults and athletes. Exercise stresses important body functions where micronutrients are required. Additionally, athletes often restrict calories and certain food groups, which may potentially lead to deficiencies of essential micronutrients. Research indicates the most common micronutrient deficiencies include:

- Iron deficiency: can impair muscle function and compromise athletic performance.
- Vitamin D deficiency: can result in decreased bone strength and reduced muscle metabolic function.
- Calcium deficiency: can impair the repair of bone tissue, decrease regulation of muscle contraction, and reduce nerve conduction.

Roles of a Sports Dietitian

Athletes and active adults are seeking guidance from sports professionals to enhance their athletic performance. Sports dietitians are increasingly hired to develop nutrition and fluid programs catered to the individual athlete or teams. A unique credential has been created for sports nutrition professionals: Board Certified Specialist in Sports Dietetics (CSSD). Sports dietitians should have knowledge in the following areas:

- Clinical nutrition,
- Nutrition science,
- Exercise physiology,

- Evidence-based research,
- Safe and effective nutrition assessments,
- Sports nutrition guidance,
- Counseling for health and athletic performance,
- Medical nutrition therapy,
- Design and management of effective nutrition strategies and
- Effective nutrition programming for health, fitness, and optimal physical performance.

Malnutrition

Malnutrition is a state of nutrition in which a deficiency or excess (or imbalance) of energy, protein and other nutrients causes measurable adverse effects on tissue / body form (body shape, size and composition) and function and clinical outcome.

Symptoms of Malnutrition

Malnutrition can often be very difficult to recognise, particularly in patients who are overweight or obese to start with. Malnutrition can happen very gradually, which can make it very difficult to spot in the early stages. Some of the symptoms and signs to watch out for include:

- Loss of appetite,
- Weight loss – clothes, rings, jewellery, dentures may become loose,
- Tiredness, loss of energy,
- Reduced ability to perform normal tasks,
- Reduced physical performance – for example, not being able to walk as far or as fast as usual,
- Altered mood – malnutrition can be associated with lethargy and depression,
- Poor concentration,
- Poor growth in children.

People who are at the risk of malnutrition:

- Older people over the age of 65, particularly if they are living in a care home or nursing home or have been admitted to hospital.
- People with long-term conditions, such as diabetes, kidney disease, chronic lung disease.
- People with chronic progressive conditions – for example, dementia or cancer.
- People who abuse drugs or alcohol.

There are also social factors that can increase the risk of malnutrition including:

- Poverty.
- Social isolation.
- Cultural norms – for example, hospitals and care homes may not always provide food that meets particular religious or cultural needs and so increase the risk of malnutrition whilst a person is away from their normal environment.

Physical factors can also increase the risk of malnutrition. For example:

- Eating may be difficult because of a painful mouth or teeth.
- Swallowing may be more difficult (a stroke can affect swallowing) or painful.
- Losing your sense of smell or taste may affect your appetite.
- Being unable to cook for yourself may result in reduced food intake.
- Limited mobility or lack of transport may make it difficult to get food.

It is also important to realise that if an older person is less able to feed themselves and becomes malnourished, this will make them more susceptible to disease, which in turn will make their nutritional state worse and impair recovery. The Malnutrition Carousel below describes this downward vicious spiral.

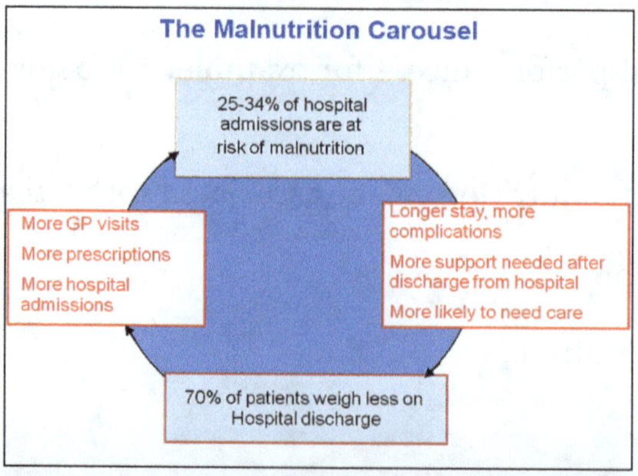

Consequences of Malnutrition

Malnutrition affects every system in the body and always results in increased vulnerability to illness, increased complications and in very extreme cases even death.

1. Immune system: Reduced ability to fight infection.

2. Muscles:

- Inactivity and reduced ability to work, shop, cook and self-care,
- Inactivity may also lead to pressure ulcers and blood clots,
- Falls,
- Reduced ability to cough may predispose to chest infections and pneumonia and
- Heart failure.

Impaired wound Healing

1. Kidneys: Inability to regulate salt and fluid can lead to over-hydration or dehydration.

2. Brain: Malnutrition causes apathy, depression, introversion, self-neglect and deterioration in social interactions.

3. Reproduction: Malnutrition reduces fertility and if present during pregnancy can predispose to problems with diabetes, heart disease and stroke in the baby in later life.

4. Impaired temperature regulation: This can lead to hypothermia.

Consequences of malnutrition in children and adolescents:

- Growth failure and stunting,
- Delayed sexual development,
- Reduced muscle mass and strength,
- Impaired intellectual development,
- Rickets and
- Increased lifetime risk of osteoporosis.

Consequences of specific micronutrient deficiencies:

- Iron deficiency can cause anaemia,

- Zinc deficiency causes skin rashes and decreased ability to fight infection,
- Vitamin B12 deficiency can cause anaemia and problems with nerves,
- Vitamin D deficiency causes rickets in children and osteomalacia in adults,
- Vitamin C deficiency causes scurvy and
- Vitamin A deficiency causes night blindness.

Detection of Malnutrition

The best way to detect malnutrition is by the use of malnutrition screening tools, such as the 'Malnutrition Universal Screening Tool' ('MUST').This tool consists of three parts:

- Body Mass Index (BMI) –This is calculated from an individual's weight and height. A BMI of less than 18.5kg/m² suggests a significant risk of malnutrition.
- A history of recent weight loss that has happened without any intention to lose weight. The unintentional loss of more than 10% of normal body weight in the last 3 -6 months suggests a significant risk of malnutrition.
- An "acute disease effect" associated with being acutely ill and unable to eat for more than five days.

This tool assesses patients as being at low, medium or high risk of malnutrition and guides the user to develop individualised care plans for treatment if required and further monitoring.

Treatment of Malnutrition

Recognising the problem is the most important first step. Once individuals and those involved in their care are aware of the problem, often simple measures to increase food intake may be enough to reverse the downward cycle. We know for example that giving nutritional supplements to malnourished patients reduces complications such as wound breakdown by 70% and death by 40%.

Once an individual has been assessed as being at risk of malnutrition it is always necessary to assess the problem in more detail and identify any other factors that are contributing to the problem. Treatment should always be tailored to the needs of the individual, but in general, if a person is able to eat and does not have a diminished appetite, then the first step would to encourage this with a "Food first" approach. This may be in the form of advice on meals, snacks, nourishing drinks and food fortification, but should include setting goals of treatment and a plan for monitoring to ensure that these goals are met.

If simple measures are not working or where the patient has a reduced appetite, then an assessment and support from a dietitian may be needed. In addition to fortifying food and increasing what you eat, there are many different oral nutritional supplements. These should usually only be used under the supervision of a dietitian or doctor. It is also possible that you may need to take a vitamin and mineral supplement – but only if advised to do so by the professional treating you.

For patients who are unable to eat, nutrition can be provided by tube feeding – either into the gut (Enteral) or directly into the bloodstream via a vein (Parenteral).

Enteral Tube Feeding (Enteral Nutrition/EN)

The commonest type of enteral tube feeding uses a tube that is passed through the nose and down into the stomach (a nasogastric tube). This is usually for short term feeding (less than 4 weeks) to provide nutritional support as a patient recovers from illness.

For longer term feeding into the stomach, a tube is usually placed through the abdomen directly into the stomach (a PEG tube, or Percutaneous Gastrostomy tube).

If it is not possible to use the stomach, it is also possible to place tubes into the jejunum (the first part of the small intestine or small bowel). These can either be nasojejunal tubes (short –term) or jejunostomy tubes which are place through the abdominal wall directly (long-term).

Parenteral Nutrition (PN)

If it is not possible to use your gut for nutrition (for example in patients who have lost part of their gut or in whom the gut does not work properly to be able to absorb nutrients) then nutrients can be given directly into the blood stream. The sterile feed is given through a small tube (catheter) placed in a vein and is tailored to ensure that you are given all the nutrients that your body needs. For most patients this is done whilst they are in hospital for no more than a few weeks as they recover from illness. However for some patients, this is their only means of nutrition and they learn to do this themselves at home (Home Parenteral Nutrition or HPN).

Types of Malnutrition

Malnutrition is a group of conditions in children and adults generally related to poor quality or insufficient quantity of nutrient intake, absorption, or utilization.

There are two major types of malnutrition:

- Protein-energy malnutrition -Resulting from deficiencies in any or all nutrients.
- Micronutrient deficiency diseases -Resulting from a deficiency of specific micronutrients.

Protein-energy Malnutrition

There are three types of protein-energy malnutrition in children:

Type	Appearance	Cause
Acute malnutrition	Wasting or thinness	Acute inadequate nutrition leading to rapid weight loss or failure to gain weight normally.
Chronic malnutrition	Stunting or shortness	Inadequate nutrition over long period of time leading to failure of linear growth.
Acute and chronic malnutrition	Underweight	A combination measure, therefore, it could occur as a result of wasting, stunting, or both.

These forms of protein-energy malnutrition in children can be pictured like this:

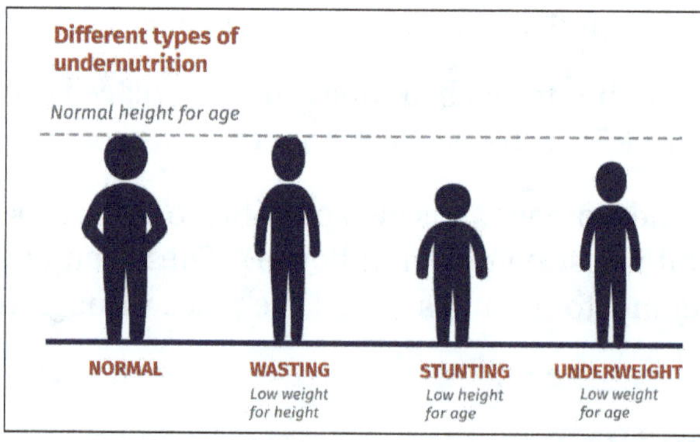

Wasting and stunting are very different forms of malnutrition. Stunting is chronic and its causative factors are poorly understood. Stunting usually does not pose an immediate threat to life and is relatively common in many populations in less-developed countries. This is not to say that it is unimportant, just less important than wasting in humanitarian emergencies. Wasting results from an acute shortage of food, is reversible with refeeding, and has a relatively high mortality rate. For these reasons, wasting is the highest priority form of malnutrition in humanitarian emergencies.

Nutritional Disease

Nutritional disease is any of the nutrient-related diseases and conditions that cause illness in humans. Nutritional diseases also include developmental abnormalities that can be prevented by diet, hereditary metabolic disorders that respond to dietary treatment, the interaction of foods and nutrients with drugs, food allergies and intolerances, and potential hazards in the food supply.

Vitamin A

Vitamin A deficiency is the leading cause of preventable blindness. Night blindness is an early sign of vitamin A deficiency, followed by abnormal dryness of the eye and ultimately scarring of the cornea, a condition known as xerophthalmia. Other symptoms include dry skin, hardening of epithelial cells elsewhere in the body (such as mucous membranes), and impaired growth and development. In many areas where vitamin A deficiency is endemic, the incidence is being reduced by giving children a single large dose of vitamin A every six months. A genetically modified form of rice containing beta-carotene, a precursor of vitamin A, has the potential to reduce greatly the incidence of vitamin A deficiency, but the use of this so-called golden rice is controversial.

Vitamin D

Vitamin D (also known as vitamin D hormone) is synthesized in the body in a series of steps, starting in the skin by the action of sunlight's ultraviolet rays on a precursor compound; thus, without adequate food sources of vitamin D, a deficiency of the vitamin can occur when exposure to sunlight is limited. Lack of vitamin D in children causes rickets, a disease characterized by inadequate mineralization of bone, growth retardation, and skeletal deformities such as bowed legs. The adult form of rickets, known as osteomalacia, results in weak muscles as well as weak bones. Inadequate vitamin D may also contribute to the thinning of bones seen in osteoporosis. Individuals with limited sun exposure (including women who completely cover their bodies for religious reasons), elderly or homebound persons, and those with dark skin, particularly those who live in northern latitudes, are at risk of vitamin D deficiency. Vitamin D is found in very few foods naturally; thus fortification of milk and other foods (e.g., margarine, cereals, and breads) with the vitamin has helped protect those populations in which sun exposure is inadequate. Supplemental vitamin D also may help protect against bone fractures in the elderly, who make and activate vitamin D less efficiently even if exposed to sunlight.

Vitamin E

Vitamin E deficiency is rare in humans, although it may develop in premature infants and in people with impaired fat absorption or metabolism. In the former, fragility of red blood cells (hemolysis) is seen; in the latter, where deficiency is more prolonged, neuromuscular dysfunction involving the spinal cord and retina may result in loss of reflexes, impaired balance and coordination, muscle weakness, and visual disturbances. No specific metabolic function has been established for vitamin E; however, it is an important part of the antioxidant system that inhibits lipid peroxidation; i.e., it protects cells and their membranes against the damaging effects of free radicals (reactive oxygen and nitrogen species) that are produced metabolically or enter the body from the environment. The requirement for vitamin E is increased with increasing consumption of polyunsaturated fatty acids. People who smoke or are subjected to air pollution may also need more of the vitamin to protect against oxidative damage to the lungs.

Vitamin K

Vitamin K is necessary for the formation of prothrombin and other blood-clotting factors in the liver, and it also plays a role in bone metabolism. A form of the vitamin is produced by bacteria in the colon and can be utilized to some degree. Vitamin K deficiency causes impaired clotting of the blood and internal bleeding, even without injury. Due to poor transport of vitamin K across the placenta, newborn infants in developed countries are routinely given the vitamin intramuscularly or orally within six hours of birth to protect against a condition known as hemorrhagic disease of the newborn. Vitamin K deficiency is rare in adults, except in syndromes with poor fat absorption, in liver disease, or during treatment with certain anticoagulant drugs, which interfere with vitamin K metabolism. Bleeding due to vitamin K deficiency may be seen in patients whose gut bacteria have been killed by antibiotics.

Thiamin

Prolonged deficiency of thiamin (vitamin B_1) results in beriberi, a disease that has been endemic in populations where white rice has been the staple. Thiamin deficiency is still seen in areas where white rice or flour constitutes the bulk of the diet and thiamin lost in milling is not replaced through enrichment. Symptoms of the form known as dry beriberi include loss of appetite, confusion and other mental symptoms, muscle weakness, painful calf muscles, poor coordination, tingling and paralysis. In wet beriberi there is edema and the possibility of an enlarged heart and heart failure. Thiamin deficiency can also occur in populations eating large quantities of raw fish harbouring intestinal microbes that contain the enzyme thiaminase. In the developed world, thiamin deficiency is linked primarily to chronic alcoholism with poor diet, manifesting as Wernicke-Korsakoff syndrome, a condition with rapid eye movements, loss of muscle coordination, mental confusion, and memory loss.

Riboflavin

Riboflavin (vitamin B_2) deficiency, known as ariboflavinosis, is unlikely without the simultaneous deficiency of other nutrients. After several months of riboflavin deprivation, symptoms include cracks in the skin at the corners of the mouth, fissures of the lips, and an inflamed, magenta-coloured tongue. Because riboflavin is readily destroyed by ultraviolet light, jaundiced infants who are treated with light therapy are administered the vitamin. Milk, milk products, and cereals, major sources of riboflavin in the diet, are packaged to prevent exposure to light.

Niacin

Symptoms of pellagra develop about two months after niacin is withdrawn from the diet. Pellagra is characterized by the so-called three Ds—diarrhea, dermatitis, and dementia—and, if it is allowed to progress untreated, death ensues. The niacin in corn and other cereal grains is largely in bound form, unable to be absorbed well. Soaking corn in lime water, as practiced by Native American populations for centuries, frees bound niacin and thus protects against pellagra. In addition, unlike other cereals, corn is low in the amino acid tryptophan, which can be converted in part to niacin. Sufficient high-quality protein (containing tryptophan) in the diet can protect against niacin deficiency even if intake of niacin itself is inadequate.

Vitamin B_6

Vitamin B_6 (pyridoxine and related compounds) is essential in protein metabolism, the synthesis of neurotransmitters, and other critical functions in the body. Deficiency symptoms include dermatitis, microcytic hypochromic anemia (small, pale red blood cells), impaired immune function, depression, confusion, and convulsions. Although full-blown vitamin B_6 deficiency is rare, marginal inadequacy is more widespread, especially among the elderly, who may have a reduced ability to absorb the vitamin. People with alcoholism, especially those with the liver diseases cirrhosis and hepatitis, are at risk of deficiency. A number of drugs, including the tuberculosis drug isoniazid, interfere with vitamin B_6 metabolism.

Folic Acid

Vitamin B_{12} and folic acid (folate) are two B vitamins with many closely related functions, notably participation in DNA synthesis. As a result, people with deficiencies of either vitamin show many of the same symptoms, such as weakness and fatigue due to megaloblastic anemia, a condition in which red blood cells, lacking sufficient DNA for cell division, are large and immature. Deficiency of folic acid also causes disruption of cell division along the gastrointestinal tract, which results in persistent diarrhea, and impaired synthesis of white blood cells and platelets. Inadequate intake of the vitamin in early pregnancy may cause neural tube defects in the fetus. Thus, women capable of becoming pregnant are advised to take 400 micrograms (μg) of folic acid daily from supplements, fortified foods (such as fortified cereals), or both—in addition to consuming foods rich in folic acid such as fresh fruits and vegetables (especially leafy greens) and legumes. The cancer drug methotrexate interferes with folic acid metabolism, causing side effects such as hair loss and diarrhea. Folic acid deficiency may also result from heavy use of alcohol, which interferes with absorption of the vitamin.

Vitamin B_{12}

Deficiency of vitamin B_{12} (cobalamin), like folic acid, results in megaloblastic anemia (large, immature red blood cells), due to interference with normal DNA synthesis. Additionally, vitamin B_{12} maintains the myelin sheath that protects nerve fibres; therefore, an untreated deficiency of the vitamin can result in nerve degeneration and eventually paralysis. Large amounts of folic acid (over 1,000 μg per day) may conceal, and possibly even exacerbate, an underlying vitamin B_{12} deficiency. Only animal foods are reliable sources of vitamin B_{12}. Vegans, who eat no foods of animal origin, are at risk of vitamin B_{12} deficiency and must obtain the vitamin through fortified food or a supplement. For people who regularly eat animal products, deficiency of the vitamin is unlikely, unless there is a defect in absorption. In order to be absorbed, vitamin B_{12} must be bound to intrinsic factor, a substance secreted by the stomach. If intrinsic factor is absent (due to an autoimmune disorder known as pernicious anemia) or if there is insufficient production of hydrochloric acid by the stomach, absorption of the vitamin will be limited. Pernicious anemia, which occurs most often in the elderly, can be treated by injections or massive oral doses (1,000 μg) of vitamin B_{12}.

Pantothenic Acid

Pantothenic acid is so widespread in foods that deficiency is unlikely under normal circumstances. Deficiency has been seen only in individuals fed semisynthetic diets deficient in the vitamin or in subjects given a pantothenic acid antagonist. Symptoms of deficiency include fatigue, irritability, sleep disturbances, abdominal distress, and neurological symptoms such as tingling in the hands. Deficiency of the vitamin was suspected during World War II when prisoners of war in Asia who exhibited "burning feet" syndrome, characterized by numbness and tingling in the toes and other neurological symptoms, responded only to the administration of pantothenic acid.

Biotin

Deficiency of biotin is rare, and this may be due in part to synthesis of the vitamin by bacteria in the colon, although the importance of this source is unclear. Biotin deficiency has been observed in people who regularly eat large quantities of raw egg white, which contains a glycoprotein (avidin) that binds biotin and prevents its absorption. A rare genetic defect that renders some infants unable to absorb a form of biotin in food can be treated with a supplement of the vitamin. Long-term use of certain anticonvulsant drugs may also impair biotin absorption. Symptoms of deficiency include skin rash, hair loss, and eventually neurological abnormalities.

Vitamin C

Vitamin C, also known as ascorbic acid, functions as a water-soluble antioxidant and as a cofactor in various enzyme systems, such as those involved in the synthesis of connective tissue components and neurotransmitters. Symptoms of scurvy, a disease caused by vitamin C deficiency, include pinpoint hemorrhages (petechiae) under the skin, bleeding gums, joint pain, and impaired wound healing. Although rare in developed countries, scurvy is seen occasionally in people consuming restricted diets, particularly those containing few fruits and vegetables, or in infants fed boiled cow's milk and no source of vitamin C. Scurvy can be prevented with relatively small quantities of vitamin C (10 milligrams [mg] per day), although recommended intakes, which aim to provide sufficient antioxidant protection, are closer to 100 mg per day. Disease states, environmental toxins, drugs, and other stresses can increase an individual's vitamin C needs. Smokers, for example, may require an additional 35 mg of the vitamin daily to maintain vitamin C levels comparable to nonsmokers.

Minerals

Iron

Iron deficiency is the most common of all nutritional deficiencies, with much of the world's population being deficient in the mineral to some degree. Young children and premenopausal women are the most vulnerable. The main function of iron is in the formation of hemoglobin, the red pigment of the blood that carries oxygen from the lungs to other tissues. Since each millilitre of blood contains 0.5 mg of iron (as a component of hemoglobin), bleeding can drain the body's iron reserves. When iron stores are depleted a condition arises known as microcytic hypochromic anemia, characterized by small red blood cells that contain less hemoglobin than normal. Symptoms of severe iron deficiency anemia include fatigue, weakness, apathy, pale skin, difficulty breathing on exertion, and low resistance to cold temperatures. During childhood, iron deficiency can affect behaviour and learning ability as well as growth and development. Severe anemia increases the risk of pregnancy complications and maternal death. Iron deficiency anemia is most common during late infancy and early childhood, when iron stores present from birth are exhausted and milk, which is poor in iron, is a primary food; during the adolescent growth spurt; and in women during the childbearing years, because of blood loss during menstruation and the additional iron needs of pregnancy. Intestinal blood loss and subsequent iron deficiency anemia in adults may also stem from ulcers, hemorrhoids, tumours, or chronic use of certain drugs such as aspirin. In developing countries, blood loss due to hookworm and other infections, coupled with inadequate dietary iron intake, exacerbates iron deficiency in both children and adults.

Iodine

Iodine deficiency disorders are the most common cause of preventable brain damage, which affects an estimated 50 million people worldwide. During pregnancy, severe iodine deficiency may impair fetal development, resulting in cretinism (irreversible mental retardation with short stature and developmental abnormalities) as well as in miscarriage and stillbirth. Other more pervasive consequences of chronic iodine deficiency include lesser cognitive and neuromuscular deficits. The ocean is a dependable source of iodine, but away from coastal areas iodine in food is variable and largely reflects the amount in the soil. In chronic iodine deficiency the thyroid gland enlarges as it attempts to trap more iodide (the form in which iodine functions in the body) from the blood for synthesis of thyroid hormones, and it eventually becomes a visible lump at the front of the neck known as a goitre. Some foods, such as cassava, millet, sweet potato, certain beans, and members of the cabbage family, contain substances known as goitrogens that interfere with thyroid hormone synthesis; these substances, which are destroyed by cooking, can be a significant factor in persons with coexisting iodine deficiency who rely on goitrogenic foods as staples.

Zinc

A constituent of numerous enzymes, zinc plays a structural role in proteins and regulates gene expression. Deficiency of the mineral was attributed to the regional diet, which was low in meat and high in legumes, unleavened breads, and whole-grain foods that contain fibre, phytic acid, and other factors that inhibit zinc absorption. Also contributing to zinc deficiency was the practice of clay eating, which interferes with the absorption of zinc, iron, and other minerals. Severe zinc deficiency has also been described in patients fed intravenous solutions inadequate in zinc and in the inherited zinc-responsive syndrome known as acrodermatitis enteropathica. Symptoms of zinc deficiency may include skin lesions, diarrhea, increased susceptibility to infections, night blindness, reduced taste and smell acuity, poor appetite, hair loss, slow wound healing, low sperm count, and impotence. Zinc is highest in protein-rich foods, especially red meat and shellfish, and zinc status may be low in protein-energy malnutrition. Even in developed countries, young children, pregnant women, the elderly, strict vegetarians, people with alcoholism, and those with malabsorption syndromes are vulnerable to zinc deficiency.

Calcium

Almost all the calcium in the body is in the bones and teeth, the skeleton serving as a reservoir for calcium needed in the blood and elsewhere. During childhood and adolescence, adequate calcium intake is critical for bone growth and calcification. A low calcium intake during childhood, and especially during the adolescent growth spurt, may predispose one to osteoporosis, a disease characterized by reduced bone mass, later in life. As bones lose density, they become fragile and unable to withstand ordinary strains; the resulting fractures, particularly of the hip, may cause incapacitation and even death. Osteoporosis is particularly common in postmenopausal women in industrial societies. Not a calcium-deficiency disease per se, osteoporosis is strongly influenced by heredity; risk of the disease can be lessened by ensuring adequate calcium intake throughout life and engaging in regular weight-bearing exercise. Sufficient calcium intake in the immediate postmenopausal years does appear to slow bone loss, although not to the same extent as do bone-conserving drugs.

Fluoride

Fluoride also contributes to the mineralization of bones and teeth and protects against tooth decay. In areas where fluoride levels in the drinking water are low, prescription fluoride supplements are recommended for children older than six months of age; dentists also may apply fluoride rinses or gels periodically to their patients' teeth. Fluoridated toothpastes are an important source of fluoride for children and also for adults, who continue to benefit from fluoride intake.

Sodium

Sodium is usually provided in ample amounts by food, even without added table salt (sodium chloride). Furthermore, the body's sodium-conservation mechanisms are highly developed, and thus sodium deficiency is rare, even for those on low-sodium diets. Sodium depletion may occur during prolonged heavy sweating, vomiting, or diarrhea or in the case of kidney disease. Symptoms of hyponatremia, or low blood sodium, include muscle cramps, nausea, dizziness, weakness, and eventually shock and coma. After prolonged high-intensity exertion in the heat, sodium balance can be restored by drinking beverages containing sodium and glucose (so-called sports drinks) and by eating salted food. Drinking a litre of water containing two millilitres (one-third teaspoon) of table salt also should suffice.

Chloride is lost from the body under conditions that parallel those of sodium loss. Severe chloride depletion results in a condition known as metabolic alkalosis (excess alkalinity in body fluids).

Potassium

Potassium is widely distributed in foods and is rarely deficient in the diet. However, some diuretics used in the treatment of hypertension deplete potassium. The mineral is also lost during sustained vomiting or diarrhea or with chronic use of laxatives. Symptoms of potassium deficiency include weakness, loss of appetite, muscle cramps, and confusion. Severe hypokalemia (low blood potassium) may result in cardiac arrhythmias. Potassium-rich foods, such as bananas or oranges, can help replace losses of the mineral, as can potassium chloride supplements, which should be taken only under medical supervision.

References

- Introduction-to-nutrition: healthengine.com.au, Retrieved 28 February, 2019
- Herbivores, nutrition, science: britannica.com, Retrieved 26 June, 2019
- Human-nutrition, science: britannica.com, Retrieved 6 April, 2019
- Fitness-sports-nutrition: verywellfit.com, Retrieved 22 January, 2019
- Introduction-to-malnutrition, malnutrition-undernutrition: bapen.org.uk, Retrieved 2 May, 2019
- Nutritional-disease, science: britannica.com, Retrieved 4 March, 2019

Chapter 3

Essential Nutrients

The nutrients are broadly classified into two categories, namely, micronutrients and macronutrients. Some of the micronutrients are vitamins and minerals while carbohydrates, proteins and fats fall under macronutrients. The topics elaborated in this chapter will help in gaining a better perspective about these different types of essential nutrients.

Essential nutrients are compounds that the body can't make or can't make in sufficient quantity. According to the World Health Organization, these nutrients must come from food, and they're vital for disease prevention, growth, and good health.

While there are many essential nutrients, they can be broken into two categories: macronutrients and micronutrients.

Macronutrients are eaten in large amounts and include the primary building blocks of your diet — protein, carbohydrates, and fat — which provide your body with energy.

Vitamins and minerals are micronutrients, and small doses go a long way. There are six main groups of essential micronutrients and macronutrients.

Carbohydrate

Carbohydrate is the class of naturally occurring compounds and derivatives formed from them. Carbohydrates are probably the most abundant and widespread organic substances in nature, and they are essential constituents of all living things. Carbohydrates are formed by green plants from carbon dioxide and water during the process of photosynthesis. Carbohydrates serve as energy sources and as essential structural components in organisms; in addition, part of the structure of nucleic acids, which contain genetic information, consists of carbohydrate.

Structural Arrangements and Properties

Stereoisomerism

Studies by German chemist Emil Fischer showed that carbohydrates, such as fructose and glucose, with the same molecular formulas but with different structural arrangements and properties (i.e., isomers) can be formed by relatively simple variations of their spatial, or geometric, arrangements. This type of isomerism, which is called stereoisomerism, exists in all biological systems. Among carbohydrates, the simplest example is provided by the three-carbon aldose sugar glyceraldehyde. There is no way by which the structures of the two isomers of glyceraldehyde, which can be distinguished by the so-called Fischer projection formulas, can be made identical, excluding breaking and reforming the linkages, or bonds, of the hydrogen (-H) and hydroxyl (-OH) groups attached to the carbon at position 2. The isomers are, in fact, mirror images akin to right and left hands; the term enantiomorphism is frequently employed for such isomerism. The chemical and physical properties of enantiomers are identical except for the property of optical rotation.

Optical rotation is the rotation of the plane of polarized light. Polarized light is light that has been separated into two beams that vibrate at right angles to each other; solutions of substances that rotate the plane of polarization are said to be optically active, and the degree of rotation is called the optical rotation of the solution. In the case of the isomers of glyceraldehyde, the magnitudes of the optical rotation are the same, but the direction in which the light is rotated-generally designated as plus, or d for dextrorotatory (to the right), or as minus, or l for levorotatory (to the left)-is opposite; i.e., a solution of D-(d)-glyceraldehyde causes the plane of polarized light to rotate to the right, and a solution of L-(l)-glyceraldehyde rotates the plane of polarized light to the left. Fischer projection formulas for the two isomers of glyceraldehyde are given below.

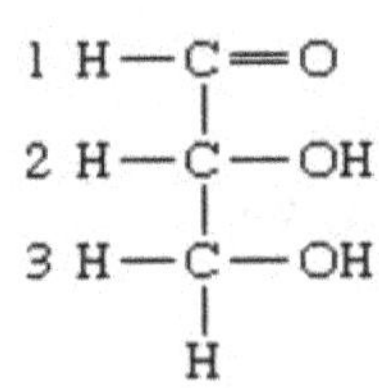
D-(*d*)-glyceraldehyde

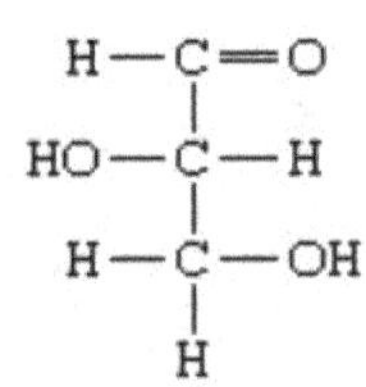
L-(*l*)-glyceraldehyde

Configuration

Molecules, such as the isomers of glyceraldehyde-the atoms of which can have different structural arrangements-are known as asymmetrical molecules. The number of possible structural arrangements for an asymmetrical molecule depends on the number of centres of asymmetry; i.e., for n (any given number of) centres of asymmetry, 2^n different isomers of a molecule are possible. An asymmetrical centre in the case of carbon is defined as a carbon atom to which four different groups are attached. In the three-carbon aldose sugar, glyceraldehyde, the asymmetrical centre is located at the central carbon atom.

(1) H—C=O, (2) H—, (3) —OH, and (4) H—C—OH.
H

The position of the hydroxyl group (-OH) attached to the central carbon atom—i.e., whether -OH projects from the left or the right—determines whether the molecule rotates the plane of polarized light to the left or to the right. Since glyceraldehyde has one asymmetrical centre, n is one in the relationship 2^n, and there thus are two possible glyceraldehyde isomers. Sugars containing four carbon atoms have two asymmetrical centres; hence, there are four possible isomers (2^2). Similarly, sugars with five carbon atoms have three asymmetrical centres and thus have eight possible isomers (2^3). Keto sugars have one less asymmetrical centre for a given number of carbon atoms than do aldehyde sugars.

A convention of nomenclature states that the form of glyceraldehyde whose asymmetrical carbon atom has a hydroxyl group projecting to the right is designated as of the D-configuration; that form, whose asymmetrical carbon atom has a hydroxyl group projecting to the left, is designated as L. All sugars that can be derived from D-glyceraldehyde—i.e., hydroxyl group attached to the asymmetrical carbon atom most remote from the aldehyde or keto end of the molecule projects to the right—are said to be of the D-configuration; those sugars derived from L-glyceraldehyde are said to be of the L-configuration.

aldehydo group (H>C=O)—of the D-configuration.

Representative disaccharides and oligosaccharides			
Common name	Component sugars	Linkages	Sources
Cellobiose	Glucose, glucose	B1 → 4*	Hydrolysis of cellulose
Gentiobiose	Glucose, glucose	B1 → 6	Plant glycosides, amygdalin
Isomaltose	Glucose, glucose	A1 → 6	Hydrolysis of glycogen, amylopectin
Raffinose**	Galactose, glucose, fructose	A1 → 6, α1 → 2	Sugarcane, beets, seeds
Stachyose**	Galactose, galactose, glucose, fructose	A1 → 6, α1 → 6, α1 → 2	Soybeans, jasmine, twigs, lentils
*The linkage joins carbon atom 1 (in the β configuration) of one glucose molecule and carbon atom 4 of the second glucose molecule; the linkage may also be abbreviated β-1, 4.			
**Raffinose and stachyose are galactosyl sucroses.			

The configurational notation D or L is independent of the sign of the optical rotation of a sugar in solution. It is common, therefore, to designate both, as, for example, D-(l)-fructose or D-(d)-glucose; i.e., both have a D-configuration at the centre of asymmetry most remote from the aldehyde end (in glucose) or keto end (in fructose) of the molecule, but fructose is levorotatory and glucose is dextrorotatory—hence the latter has been given the alternative name dextrose. Although the initial assignments of configuration for the glyceraldehydes were made on purely arbitrary grounds, studies that were carried out nearly half a century later established them as correct in an absolute spatial sense. In biological systems, only the D or L form may be utilized.

When more than one asymmetrical centre is present in a molecule, as is the case with sugars having four or more carbon atoms, a series of DL pairs exists, and they are functionally, physically, and chemically distinct. Thus, although D-xylose and D-lyxose both have five carbon atoms and are of the D-configuration, the spatial arrangement of the asymmetrical centres (at carbon atoms 2, 3, and 4) is such that they are not mirror images.

Hemiacetal and Hemiketal Forms

Although optical rotation has been one of the most frequently determined characteristics of carbohydrates, the rotational behaviour of freshly prepared solutions of many sugars differs from that of solutions that have been allowed to stand. This phenomenon, known as mutarotation, is demonstrable even with apparently identical sugars and is caused by a type of stereoisomerism involving formation of an asymmetrical centre at the first carbon atom (aldehyde carbon) in aldoses and the second one (keto carbon) in ketoses.

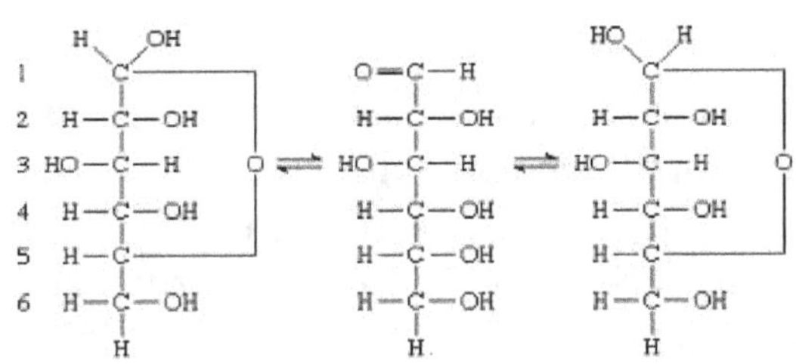

α-D-glucose (hemiacetal form) · D-glucose (linear, open-chain, or free form) · β-D-glucose (hemiacetal form)

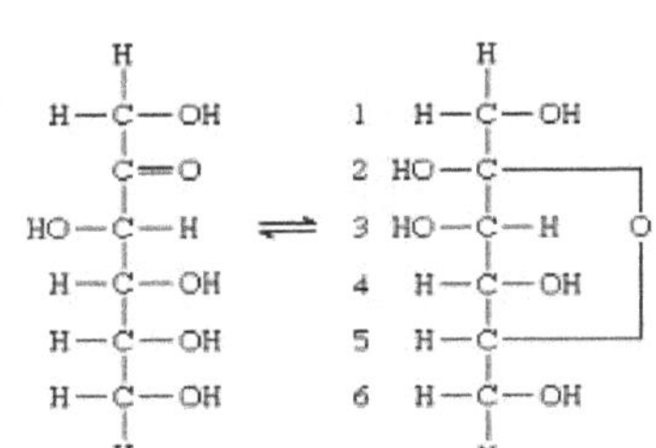

D-fructose (linear, open-chain, or free form) · α-D-fructose (hemiketal form)

Most pentose and hexose sugars, therefore, do not exist as linear, or open-chain, structures in solution but form cyclic, or ring, structures in hemiacetal or hemiketal forms, respectively. As illustrated for glucose and fructose, the cyclic structures are formed by the addition of the hydroxyl group (–OH) from either the fourth, fifth, or sixth carbon atom to the carbonyl group (>C=O) at position 1 in glucose or 2 in fructose. In the case of five-membered cyclic ketohexose or six-membered cyclic aldohexose, the cyclic forms are in equilibrium with (i.e., the rate of conversion from one form to another is stable) the open-chain structure—a free aldehyde if the solution contains glucose, a free ketone if it contains fructose; each form has a different optical rotation value. Since the forms are in equilibrium with each other, a constant value of optical rotation is measurable; the two cyclic forms represent more than 99.9 percent of the sugar in the case of a glucose solution.

By definition, the carbon atom containing the aldehyde or keto group is called the anomeric carbon atom; similarly, carbohydrate stereoisomers that differ in configuration only at this carbon atom are called anomers. When a cyclic hemiacetal or hemiketal structure forms, the structure with the new hydroxyl group projecting on the same side as that of the oxygen involved in forming the ring is called the alpha anomer; that with the hydroxyl group projecting on the opposite side from that of the oxygen ring is called the beta anomer.

alpha anomer beta anomer

The spatial arrangements of the atoms in these cyclic structures are better shown (glucose is used as an example) in the representation devised by British organic chemist Sir Norman Haworth they are still in widespread use. In the formulation the asterisk indicates the position of the anomeric carbon atom; the carbon atoms, except at position 6, usually are not labelled.

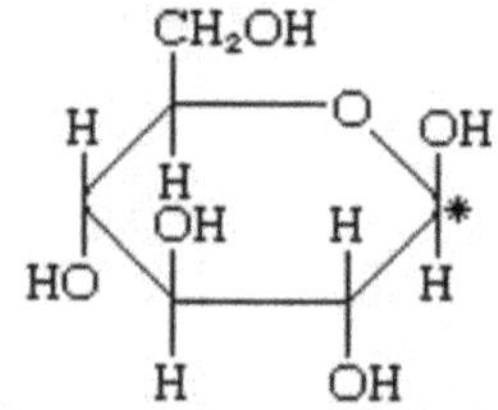

Haworth formulation of β-D-glucose

The large number of asymmetrical carbon atoms and the consequent number of possible isomers considerably complicates the structural chemistry of carbohydrates.

Classes of Carbohydrates

Monosaccharides

The most common naturally occurring monosaccharides are D-glucose, D-mannose,

D-fructose, and D-galactose among the hexoses and D-xylose and L-arabinose among the pentoses. In a special sense, D-ribose and 2-deoxy-D-ribose are ubiquitous because they form the carbohydrate component of ribonucleic acid (RNA) and deoxyribonucleic acid (DNA), respectively; these sugars are present in all cells as components of nucleic acids.

Some naturally occurring monosaccharides	
Sugar	**Sources**
L-arabinose	mesquite gum, wheat bran
D-ribose	all living cells; as component of ribonucleic acid
D-xylose	corncobs, seed hulls, straw
D-ribulose	as an intermediate in photosynthesis
2-deoxy-D-ribose	as constituent of deoxyribonucleic acid
D-galactose	lactose, agar, gum arabic, brain glycolipids
D-glucose	sucrose, cellulose, starch, glycogen
D-mannose	seeds, ivory nut
D-fructose	sucrose, artichokes, honey
L-fucose	marine algae, seaweed
L-rhamnose	poison-ivy blossom, oak bark
D-mannoheptulose	avocado
D-altroheptulose	numerous plants

D-Xylose, found in most plants in the form of a polysaccharide called xylan, is prepared from corncobs, cottonseed hulls, or straw by chemical breakdown of xylan. D-Galactose, a common constituent of both oligosaccharides and polysaccharides, also occurs in carbohydrate-containing lipids, called glycolipids, which are found in the brain and other nervous tissues of most animals. Galactose is generally prepared by acid hydrolysis (breakdown involving water) of lactose, which is composed of galactose and glucose. Since the biosynthesis of galactose in animals occurs through intermediate compounds derived directly from glucose, animals do not require galactose in the diet. In fact, in most human populations the majority of people do not retain the ability to manufacture the enzyme necessary to metabolize galactose after they reach the age of four, and many individuals possess a hereditary defect known as galactosemia and never have the ability to metabolize galactose.

D-Glucose the naturally occurring form, is found in fruits, honey, blood, and, under abnormal conditions, in urine. It is also a constituent of the two most common naturally found disaccharides, sucrose and lactose, as well as the exclusive structural unit of the polysaccharides cellulose, starch, and glycogen. Generally, D-glucose is prepared from either potato starch or cornstarch.

D-Fructose, a ketohexose, is one of the constituents of the disaccharide sucrose and is also found in uncombined form in honey, apples, and tomatoes. Fructose, generally considered the sweetest monosaccharide, is prepared by sucrose hydrolysis and is metabolized by humans.

Chemical Reactions

The reactions of the monosaccharides can be conveniently subdivided into those associated with the aldehyde or keto group and those associated with the hydroxyl groups.

The relative ease with which sugars containing a free or potentially free aldehyde or keto group can be oxidized to form products has been known for a considerable time and once was the basis for the detection of these so-called reducing sugars in a variety of sources. For many years, analyses of blood glucose and urinary glucose were carried out by a procedure involving the use of an alkaline copper compound. Because the reaction has undesirable features—extensive destruction of carbohydrate structure occurs, and the reaction is not very specific (i.e., sugars other than glucose give similar results) and does not result in the formation of readily identifiable products—blood and urinary glucose now are analyzed by using the enzyme glucose oxidase, which catalyzes the oxidation of glucose to products that include hydrogen peroxide. The hydrogen peroxide then is used to oxidize a dye present in the reaction mixture; the intensity of the colour is directly proportional to the amount of glucose initially present. The enzyme, glucose oxidase, is highly specific for β-D-glucose.

In another reaction, the aldehyde group of glucose:

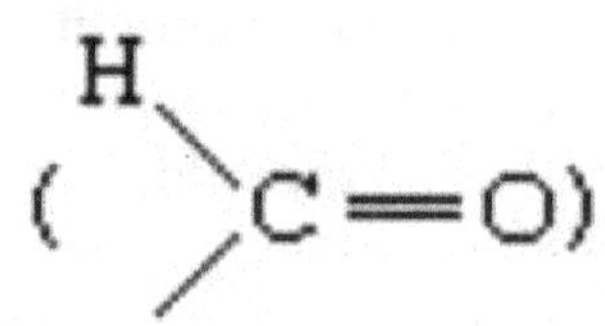

Reacts with alkaline iodine to form a class of compounds called aldonic acids. One important aldonic acid is ascorbic acid (vitamin C), an essential dietary component for humans and guinea pigs. The formation of similar acid derivatives does not occur with the keto sugars.

Either the aldehyde or the keto group of a sugar may be reduced (i.e., hydrogen added) to form an alcohol; compounds formed in this way are called alditols, or sugar alcohols. The product formed as a result of the reduction of the aldehyde carbon of D-glucose is called sorbitol (D-glucitol). D-Glucitol also is formed when L-sorbose is reduced. The reduction of mannose results in mannitol, that of galactose in dulcitol.

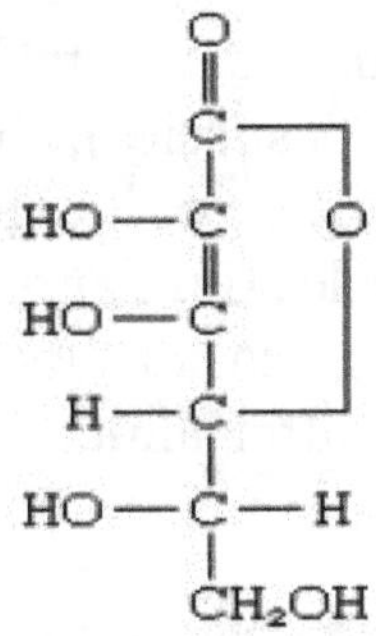

Ascorbic acid, vitamin C (L-gulonolactone-2, 3-enediol)

Sugar alcohols that are of commercial importance include sorbitol (D-glucitol), which is commonly used as a sweetening agent, and D-mannitol, which is also used as a sweetener, particularly in chewing gums, because it has a limited water solubility and remains powdery and granular on long storage.

Formation of Glycosides

The hydroxyl group that is attached to the anomeric carbon atom (i.e., the carbon containing the aldehyde or keto group) of carbohydrates in solution has unusual reactivity, and derivatives, called glycosides, can be formed; glycosides formed from glucose are called glucosides. It is not possible for equilibration between the α- and β-anomers of a glycoside in solution (i.e., mutarotation) to occur. The reaction by which a glycoside is formed involves the hydroxyl group (-OH) of the anomeric carbon atom (numbered 1) of both α and β forms of D-glucose—α and β forms of D-glucose are shown in equilibrium in the reaction sequence—and the hydroxyl group of an alcohol (methyl alcohol in the reaction sequence); methyl α-D-glucosides and β-D-glucosides are formed as products, as is water.

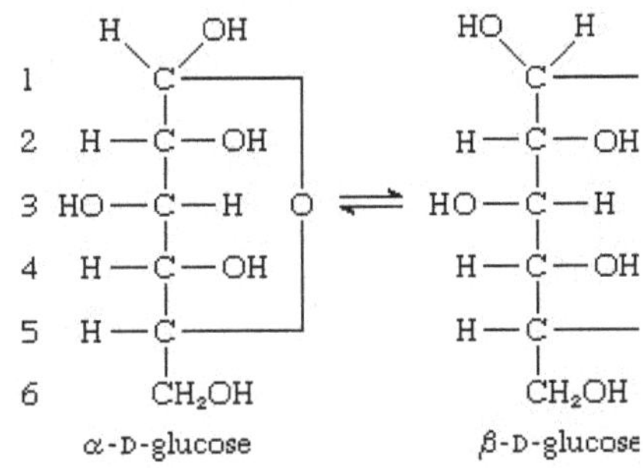

(in equilibrium in solution)

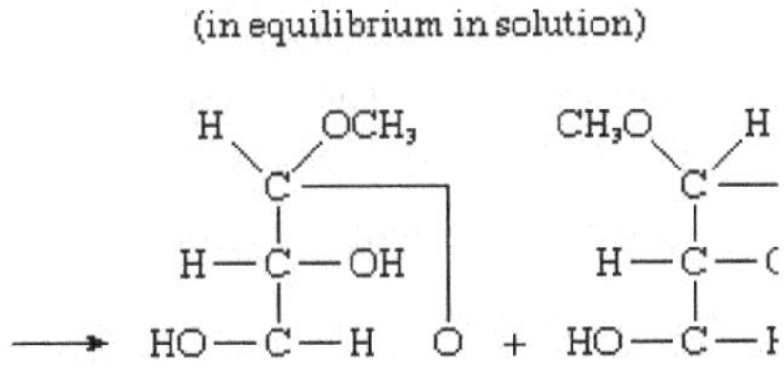

Among the wide variety of naturally occurring glycosides are a number of plant pigments, particularly those red, violet, and blue in colour; these pigments are found in flowers and consist of a pigment molecule attached to a sugar molecule, frequently glucose. Plant indican (from Indigofera species), composed of glucose and the pigment indoxyl, was important in the preparation of indigo dye before synthetic dyes became prevalent. Of a number of heart muscle stimulants that occur as glycosides, digitalis is still used. Other naturally occurring glycosides include vanillin, which is found in the vanilla bean, and amygdalin (oil of bitter almonds); a variety of glycosides found in mustard have a sulfur atom at position 1 rather than oxygen.

A number of important antibiotics are glycosides; among the best known are streptomycin and erythromycin. Glucosides-i.e., glycosides formed from glucose-in which the anomeric carbon atom (at position 1) has phosphoric acid linked to it, are extremely important biological compounds. For example, α-D-glucose-1-phosphate is an intermediate product in the biosynthesis of cellulose, starch, and glycogen; similar glycosidic phosphate derivatives of other monosaccharides participate in the formation of naturally occurring glycosides and polysaccharides.

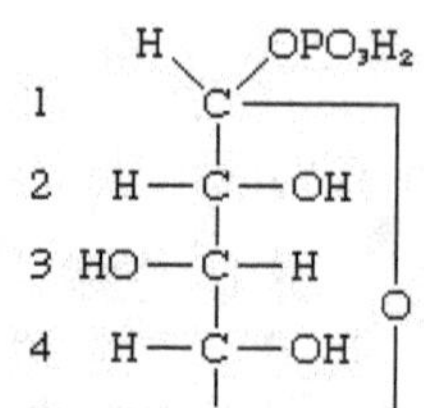

α-D-glucose-1-phosphate

The hydroxyl groups other than the one at the anomeric carbon atom can undergo a variety of reactions. Esterification, which consists of reacting the hydroxyl groups with an appropriate acidic compound, results in the formation of a class of compounds called sugar esters. Among the common ones are the sugar acetates, in which the acid is acetic acid. Esters of phosphoric acid and sulfuric acid are important biological compounds; glucose-6-phosphate, for example, plays a central role in the energy metabolism of most living cells, and D-ribulose 1,5-diphosphate is important in photosynthesis.

Formation of Methyl Ethers

Treatment of a carbohydrate with methyl iodide or similar agents under appropriate conditions results in the formation of compounds in which the hydroxyl groups are converted to methyl groups ($-CH_3$). Called methyl ethers, these compounds are employed in structural studies of oligosaccharides and polysaccharides because their formation does not break the bonds, called glycosidic bonds, that link adjacent monosaccharide units. An example is the etherification of a starch molecule carried out using methyl iodide, in which methyl groups become attached to the glucose molecules, forming a methylated segment in the starch molecule; note that the glycosidic bonds are not broken by the reaction with methyl iodide. When the methylated starch molecule then is broken down (hydrolyzed), hydroxyl groups are located at the positions in the molecule previously involved in linking one sugar molecule to another, and a methylated glucose, in this case named 2,3,6 tri-O-methyl-D-glucose, forms. The linkage positions (which are not methylated) in a complex carbohydrate can be established by analyzing the locations of the methyl groups in the monosaccharides. This technique is useful in determining the structural details of polysaccharides, particularly since the various methylated sugars are easily separated by techniques involving gas chromatography, in which a moving gas stream carries a mixture through a column of a stationary liquid or solid, the components thus being resolved.

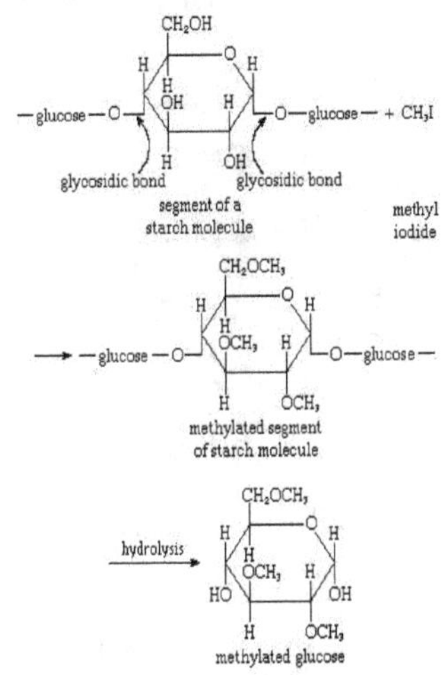

When the terminal group (CH_2OH) of a monosaccharide is oxidized chemically or biologically, a product called a uronic acid is formed. Glycosides that are derived from D-glucuronic acid (the uronic acid formed from D-glucose) and fatty substances called steroids appear in the urine of animals as normal metabolic products; in addition, foreign toxic substances are frequently converted in the liver to glucuronides before excretion in the urine. D-Glucuronic acid also is a major component of connective tissue polysaccharides, and D-galacturonic acid and D-mannuronic acid, formed from D-galactose and D-mannose, respectively, are found in several plant sources.

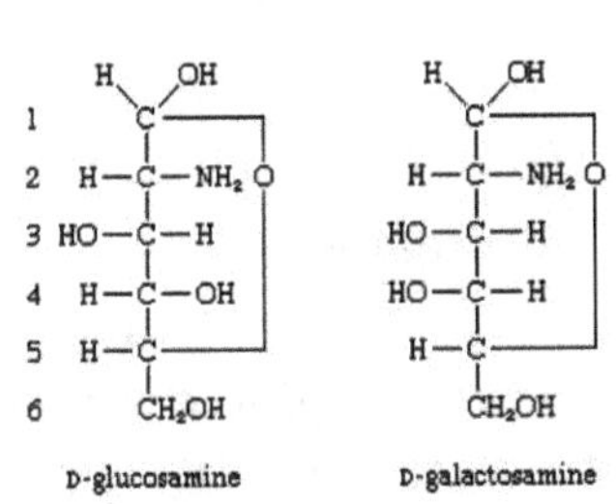

Other compounds formed from monosaccharides include those in which one hydroxyl group, usually at the carbon at position 2, is replaced by an amino group ($-NH_2$); these compounds, called amino sugars, are widely distributed in nature. The two most important ones are glucosamine (2-amino-2-deoxy-D-glucose) and galactosamine (2-amino-2-deoxy-D-galactose).

Neither amino sugar is found in the uncombined form. Both occur in animals as components of glycolipids or polysaccharides; e.g., the primary structural polysaccharide (chitin) of insect outer skeletons and various blood group substances.

In a number of naturally occurring sugars, known as deoxy sugars, the hydroxyl group at a particular position is replaced by a hydrogen atom. By far the most important representative is 2-deoxy-D-ribose, the pentose sugar found in deoxyribonucleic acid (DNA); the hydroxyl group at the carbon atom at position 2 has been replaced by a hydrogen atom.

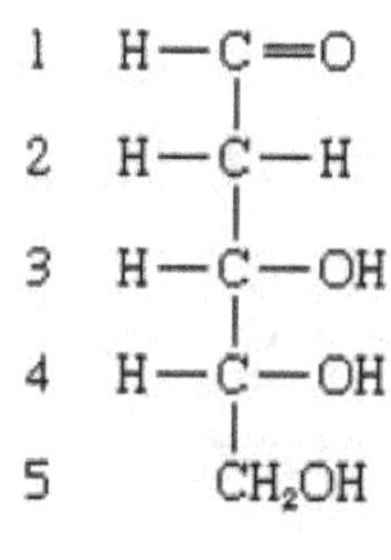

2-deoxy-D-ribose

Other naturally occurring deoxy sugars are hexoses, of which L-rhamnose (6-deoxy-L-mannose) and L-fucose (6-deoxy-L-galactose) are the most common; the latter, for example, is present in the carbohydrate portion of blood group substances and on the outer surface of red blood cells.

Disaccharides and Oligosaccharides

Disaccharides are a specialized type of glycoside in which the anomeric hydroxyl group of one sugar has combined with the hydroxyl group of a second sugar with the elimination of the elements of water. Although an enormous number of disaccharide structures are possible, only a limited number are of commercial or biological significance.

Sucrose and Trehalose

Sucrose, or common table sugar, is a major commodity worldwide. The unusual type of linkage between the two anomeric hydroxyl groups of glucose and fructose means that neither a free aldehyde group (on the glucose moiety) nor a free keto group (on the fructose moiety) is available to react unless the linkage between the monosaccharides is destroyed; for this reason, sucrose is known as a nonreducing sugar. Sucrose solutions do not exhibit mutarotation, which involves formation of an asymmetrical centre at the aldehyde or keto group. If the linkage between the monosaccharides composing sucrose is broken, the optical rotation value of sucrose changes from positive to negative; the new value reflects the composite rotation values for D-glucose, which is dextrorotatory (+52°), and D-fructose, which is levorotatory (−92°). The change in the sign of optical rotation from positive to negative is the reason sucrose is sometimes called invert sugar.

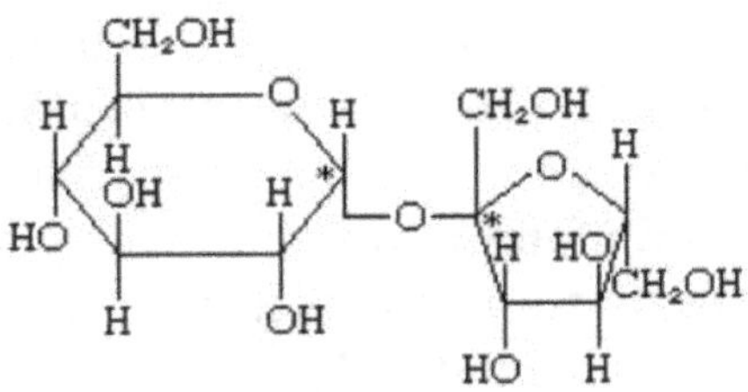

sucrose

The commercial preparation of sucrose takes advantage of the alkaline stability of the sugar, and a variety of impurities are removed from crude sugarcane extracts by treatment with alkali. After this step, syrup preparations are crystallized to form table sugar. Successive "crops" of sucrose crystals are "harvested," and the later ones are known as brown sugar. The residual syrupy material is called either cane final molasses or blackstrap molasses; both are used in the preparation of antibiotics, as sweetening agents, and in the production of alcohol by yeast fermentation. Sucrose is formed following photosynthesis in plants by a reaction in which sucrose phosphate first is formed.

The disaccharide trehalose is similar in many respects to sucrose but is much less widely distributed. It is composed of two molecules of α-D-glucose and is also a nonreducing sugar. Trehalose is present in young mushrooms and in the resurrection plant (Selaginella); it is of considerable biological interest because it is also found in the circulating fluid (hemolymph) of many insects. Since trehalose can be converted to a glucose phosphate compound by an enzyme-catalyzed reaction that does not require energy, its function in hemolymph may be to provide an immediate energy source, a role similar to that of the carbohydrate storage forms (i.e., glycogen) found in higher animals.

Lactose and Maltose

Lactose is one of the sugars (sucrose is another) found most commonly in human diets throughout the world; it constitutes about 7 percent of human milk and about 4–5 percent of the milk of mammals such as cows, goats, and sheep. Lactose consists of two aldohexoses—β-D-galactose and glucose—linked so that the aldehyde group at the anomeric carbon of glucose is free to react; i.e., lactose is a reducing sugar.

A variety of metabolic disorders related to lactose may occur in infants; in some cases, they are the result of a failure to metabolize properly the galactose portion of the molecule.

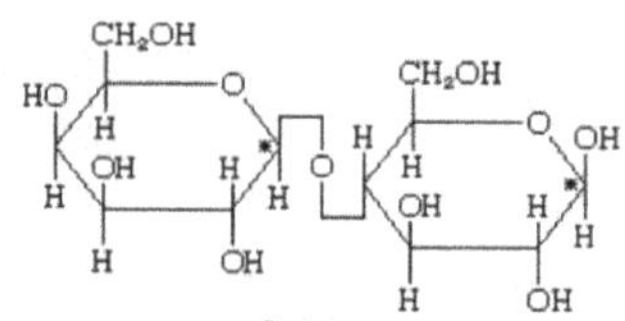

β-lactose

Although not found in uncombined form in nature, the disaccharide maltose is biologically important because it is a product of the enzymatic breakdown of starches during digestion. Maltose consists of α-D-glucose linked to a second glucose unit in such a way that maltose is a reducing sugar. Maltose, which is readily hydrolyzed to glucose and can be metabolized by animals, is employed as a sweetening agent and as a food for infants whose tolerance for lactose is limited.

Polysaccharides

Polysaccharides, or glycans, may be classified in a number of ways; the following scheme is frequently used. Homopolysaccharides are defined as polysaccharides formed from only one type of monosaccharide. Homopolysaccharides may be further subdivided into straight-chain and branched-chain representatives, depending upon the arrangement of the monosaccharide units. Heteropolysaccharides are defined as polysaccharides containing two or more different types of monosaccharides; they may also occur in both straight-chain and branched-chain forms. In general, extensive variation of linkage types does not occur within a polysaccharide structure, nor are there many polysaccharides composed of more than three or four different monosaccharides; most contain one or two.

Representative homopolysaccharides				
Homopolysaccharide	Sugar Component	Linkage	Function	Sources
Cellulose	Glucose	β, 1 → 4	Structural	Throughout plant kingdom
Amylose	Glucose	α, 1 → 4	Food storage	Starches, especially corn, potatoes, rice
Chitin	N-acetylglucosamine	β, 1 → 4	Structural	Insect and crustacean skeleton
Inulin	Fructose	β, 2 → 1	Food storage	Artichokes, chicory
Xylan	Xylose	β, 1 → 4	Structural	All land plants
Glycogen	Glucose	α, 1 → 4, 6 ← 1, α	Food storage	Liver and muscle cells of all animals
Amylopectin	Glucose	α, 1 → 4, 6 ← 1, α	Food storage	Starches, especially corn, potatoes, rice

Representative homopolysaccharides				
Dextran	Glucose	α, 1 → 6, 4 ← 1, α	Unknown	Primarily bacterial
Agar*	Galactose	α, 1 → 3	Structural	Seaweeds
*May contain sulfate groups.				

Homopolysaccharides

In general, homopolysaccharides have a well-defined chemical structure, although the molecular weight of an individual amylose or xylan molecule may vary within a particular range, depending on the source; molecules from a single source also may vary in size, because most polysaccharides are formed biologically by an enzyme-catalyzed process lacking genetic information regarding size.

The basic structural component of most plants, cellulose, is widely distributed in nature. It has been estimated that 50 billion to 100 billion tons of cellulose are synthesized yearly as a result of photosynthesis by higher plants. The proportion of cellulose to total carbohydrate found in plants may vary in various types of woods from 30 to 40 percent, and to more than 98 percent in the seed hair of the cotton plant. Cellulose, a large, linear molecule composed of 3,000 or more β-D-glucose molecules, is insoluble in water.

The chains of glucose units composing cellulose molecules are frequently aligned within the cell-wall structure of a plant to form fibre-like or crystalline arrangements. This alignment permits very tight packing of the chains and promotes their structural stability but also makes structural analysis difficult. The relationships between cellulose and other polysaccharides present in the cell wall are not well established; in addition, the presence of unusual chemical linkages or nonglucose units within the cellulose structure has not yet been established with certainty.

During the preparation of cellulose, raw plant material is treated with hot alkali; this treatment removes most of the lignin, the hemicelluloses, and the mucilaginous components. The cellulose then is processed to produce papers and fibres. The high resistance of cellulose to chemical or enzymatic breakdown is important in the manufacture of paper and cloth. Cellulose also is modified chemically for other purposes; e.g., compounds such as cellulose acetate are used in the plastics industry, in the production of photographic film, and in the rayon-fibre industry. Cellulose nitrate (nitrocellulose) is employed in the lacquer and explosives industries.

The noteworthy biological stability of cellulose is dramatically illustrated by trees, the life-span of which may be several thousand years. Enzymes capable of breaking down cellulose are generally found only among several species of bacteria and molds. The apparent ability of termites to utilize cellulose as an energy source depends on the presence in their intestinal tracts of protozoans that can break it down. Similarly, the single-celled organisms present in the rumina of sheep and cattle are responsible for the ability of these animals to utilize the cellulose present in typical grasses and other feeds.

Xylans are almost as ubiquitous as cellulose in plant cell walls and contain predominantly β-D-xylose units linked as in cellulose. Some xylans contain other sugars, such as L-arabinose, but they form branches and are not part of the main chain. Xylans are of little commercial importance.

The term starch refers to a group of plant reserve polysaccharides consisting almost exclusively of a linear component (amylose) and a branched component (amylopectin). The use of starch as an energy source by humans depends on the ability to convert it completely to individual glucose units; the process is initiated by the action of enzymes called amylases, synthesized by the salivary glands in the mouth, and continues in the intestinal tract. The primary product of amylase action is maltose, which is hydrolyzed to two component glucose units as it is absorbed through the walls of the intestine.

A characteristic reaction of the amylose component of starch is the formation with iodine of a complex compound with a characteristic blue colour. About one iodine molecule is bound for each seven or eight glucose units, and at least five times that many glucose units are needed in an amylose chain to permit the effective development of the colour.

The amylopectin component of starch is structurally similar to glycogen in that both are composed of glucose units linked together in the same way, but the distance between branch points is greater in amylopectin than in glycogen, and the former may be thought of as occupying more space per unit weight.

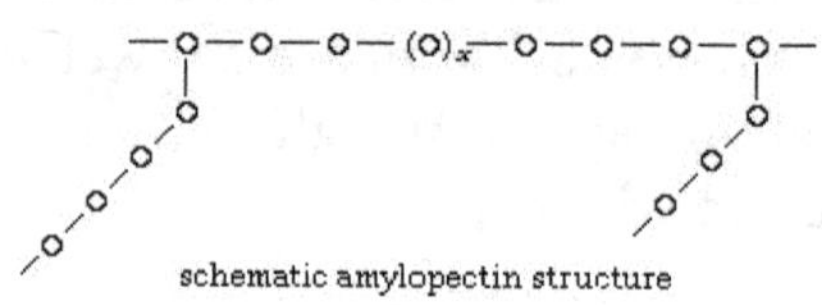

schematic amylopectin structure

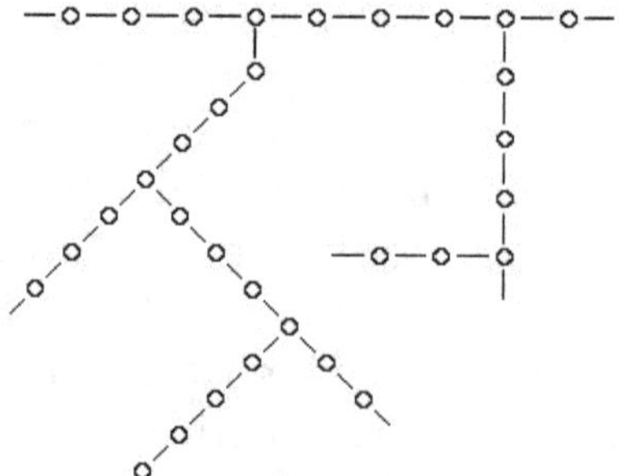

schematic glycogen structure

The applications of starches other than as foods are limited. Starches are employed in adhesive manufacture, and starch nitrate has some utility as an explosive.

Glycogen, which is found in all animal tissues, is the primary animal storage form of carbohydrate and, indirectly, of rapidly available energy. The distance between branch points in a glycogen molecule is only five or six units, which results in a compact tree-like structure. The ability of higher animals to form and break down this extensively branched structure is essential to their well-being; in conditions known as glycogen storage diseases, these activities are abnormal, and the asymmetrical glycogen molecules that are formed have severe, often fatal, consequences. Glycogen synthesis and breakdown are controlled by substances called hormones.

Large molecules—e.g., pectins and agars—composed of galactose or its uronic-acid derivative (galacturonic acid) are important because they can form gels. Pectins, which are predominantly galacturonans, are produced from citrus fruit rinds; they are used commercially in the preparation of jellies and jams. Agar is widely employed in biological laboratories as a solidifying agent for growth media for microorganisms and in the bakery industry as a gelling agent; it forms a part of the diet of people in several areas of East Asia.

Dextrans, a group of polysaccharides composed of glucose, are secreted by certain strains of bacteria as slimes. The structure of an individual dextran varies with the strain of microorganism. Dextrans can be used as plasma expanders (substitutes for whole blood) in cases of severe shock. In addition, a dextran derivative compound is employed medically as an anticoagulant for blood.

Chitin is structurally similar to cellulose, but the repeating sugar is 2-deoxy-2-acetamido-D-glucose (N-acetyl-D-glucosamine) rather than glucose.

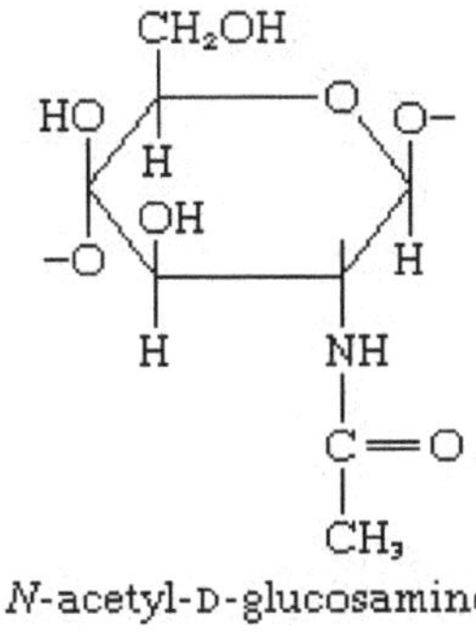

N-acetyl-D-glucosamine

Sometimes referred to as animal cellulose, chitin is the major component of the outer skeletons of insects, crustaceans, and other arthropods, as well as annelid and nematode worms, mollusks, and coelenterates. The cell walls of most fungi also are predominantly chitin, which comprises nearly 50 percent of the dry weight of some species. Since chitin is nearly as chemically inactive as cellulose and easily obtained, numerous attempts, none of which has thus far been successful, have been made to develop it commercially. The nitrogen content of the biosphere, however, is stabilized by the ability of soil microorganisms to degrade nitrogen-containing compounds such as those found in insect skeletons; these microorganisms convert the nitrogen in complex molecules to a form usable by plants. If such microorganisms did not exist, much of the organic nitrogen present in natural materials would be unavailable to plants.

Heteropolysaccharides

In general, heteropolysaccharides (heteroglycans) contain two or more different monosaccharide units. Although a few representatives contain three or more different monosaccharides, most naturally occurring heteroglycans contain only two different ones and are closely associated with lipid or protein. The complex nature of these substances has made detailed structural studies extremely difficult. The major heteropolysaccharides include the connective-tissue polysaccharides, the blood group substances, glycoproteins (combinations of carbohydrates and proteins) such as gamma globulin, and glycolipids (combinations of carbohydrates and lipids), particularly those found in the central nervous system of animals and in a wide variety of plant gums.

Representative heteropolysaccharides			
Heteropolysaccharide	Component Sugars	Functions	Fistribution
Hyaluronic acid	D-glucuronic acid and *N*-acetyl-D-glucosamine	Lubricant, shock absorber, water binding	Connective tissue, skin
Chondroitin-4-sulfate*	D-glucuronic acid and *N*-acetyl-D-galactosamine-4-*O*-sulfate	Calcium accumulation, cartilage and bone formation	Cartilage
Heparin*	D-glucuronic acid, *L*-iduronic acid, *N*-sulfo-D-glucosamine	Anticoagulant	Mast cells, blood
Gamma globulin*	*N*-acetyl-hexosamine, D-mannose, D-galactose	Antibody	Blood
Blood group substance*	D-glucosamine, D-galactosamine, *L*-fucose, D-galactose	Blood group specificity	Cell surfaces, especially red blood cells
*Covalently linked to protein; the proportion of protein to carbohydrate in such complex molecules varies from about 10% protein in the case of chondroitin-4-sulfate to better than 95% for gamma globulin.			

The most important heteropolysaccharides are found in the connective tissues of all animals and include a group of large molecules that vary in size, shape, and interaction with other body substances. They have a structural role, and the structures of individual connective-tissue polysaccharides are related to specific animal functions; hyaluronic acid, for example, the major component of joint fluid in animals, functions as a lubricating agent and shock absorber.

The connective-tissue heteropolysaccharides contain acidic groups (uronic acids or sulfate groups) and can bind both water and inorganic metal ions. They can also play a role in other physiological functions; e.g., in the accumulation of calcium before bone formation. Ion-binding ability also appears to be related to the anticoagulant activity of the heteropolysaccharide heparin.

The size of the carbohydrate portion of glycoproteins such as gamma globulin or hen-egg albumin is usually between five and 10 monosaccharide units; several such units occur in some glycoprotein molecules. The function of the carbohydrate component has not yet been established except for glycoproteins associated with cell surfaces; in this case, they appear to act as antigenic determinants—i.e., they are capable of inducing the formation of specific antibodies.

Preparation and Analysis

In general, monosaccharides are prepared by breakdown with acids of the polysaccharides in which they occur. Sugars usually are difficult to obtain in crystalline form, and the crystallization process usually is begun by "seeding" a concentrated solution of the sugar with crystals. The techniques employed for separation of monosaccharides depend to some extent on their physical and chemical properties; chromatographic procedures are often used.

Oligosaccharides and polysaccharides are prepared from natural sources by techniques that take advantage of size, alkaline stability, or some combination of these and other properties of the molecule of interest. It should be noted that preparation of an oligosaccharide or polysaccharide usually results in a range of molecular sizes of the desired molecule. The purity of a carbohydrate preparation, which is frequently based on an analysis of its composition, is more easily established for monosaccharides and disaccharides than for large, insoluble molecules such as cellulose.

Analytical Techniques

A variety of organic chemical analytical techniques are generally applicable to studies involving carbohydrates. Optical rotation, for example, once was frequently used to characterize carbohydrates. The ability to measure the rotation of the plane of polarized light transmitted through a solution containing a carbohydrate depends on finding a suitable solvent; water usually is used, with light at a wavelength of 589 mμ (millimicrons). Optical rotation is no longer widely used to characterize monosaccharides. The magnitude and sign of the optical rotation of glycosides, however, is useful in assigning configuration (α or β) to the hydroxyl group at the anomeric centre; glycosides of the α-configuration generally have rotations of higher magnitude than do the same glycosides of the β-configuration. Optical rotation is not a completely additive property; a trisaccharide composed of three glucose residues, for example, does not have a rotation three times that of one glucose molecule. Sugar alcohols cannot form ring structures; their rotation values are extremely small, suggesting a relationship between ring structure and the ability of a carbohydrate to rotate the plane of polarized light. Certain types of reactions (e.g., glycoside hydrolysis) can be monitored by measuring the change in optical rotation as a function of time. This technique is frequently used to examine the breakdown of disaccharides or oligosaccharides to monosaccharide units, especially if a large change in the net optical rotation may be expected, as occurs in the hydrolysis of sucrose.

Spectroscopic Techniques

Several other optical techniques used in chemistry have been applied to the analysis of carbohydrates. Infrared spectroscopy, used to measure vibrational and rotational excitation of molecules, and nuclear magnetic-resonance spectroscopy, which measures the excitation of certain components of molecules in a magnetic field induced by radio-frequency radiation, are valuable, although the similarity of the functional groups (i.e., the hydroxyl groups) limits use of the former technique for most sugars. Proton magnetic-resonance spectroscopy, nuclear magnetic resonance applied to protons (H atoms), is employed to identify the relative spatial arrangements of individual hydrogen atoms in a molecule. When they are precisely placed, the corresponding positions of the hydroxyl groups attached to the same carbon atom can be deduced. An extension of this technique utilizes the resonance spectroscopy of carbon-13, a nonradioactive isotope of carbon, so that ring structures can be established with great accuracy. Both the proton and carbon magnetic resonance methods are best applied to monosaccharides; they are less valuable in studying polysaccharides because an individual hydrogen atom in a large molecule is too small for accurate detection.

Identification of Subunits

The study of polysaccharide structure usually focuses on the chemical composition, the linkage between the monosaccharide units, and the size and shape of the molecule. The size and shape of a polysaccharide can be ascertained by techniques that are usually applied to large molecules; e.g., the most accurate molecular weight determination measures the sedimentation properties of the molecule in an applied gravitational field (e.g., the rate at which a solid material is deposited from a state of suspension or solution in a liquid). Indications of the shape of polysaccharide molecules in solution are obtained from viscosity measurements, in which the resistance of the molecules to flow (viscosity) is equated with the end-to-end length of the molecule; the viscosity of hyaluronic acid, for example, shows a marked dependence on both concentration of the acid and the salt content of the solution, and, under conditions approximating those found in biological systems, a hyaluronic acid molecule may be thought of as occupying a great deal of space. Alternatively, the compact nature of a glycogen molecule of molecular weight equal to that of a molecule of hyaluronic acid results in its accommodation to a much smaller space than the latter molecule.

The identification of sugars in a mixture resulting from the hydrolytic breakdown of a heteropolysaccharide is most often carried out by chromatography of the mixture on paper, silica gel, or cellulose. Ready separations can be achieved between pentoses, hexoses and, for example, deoxy sugars; closely related compounds such as D-glucose and D-galactose also can be separated using chromatographic techniques. The linkage positions in polysaccharides are usually determined using the methylation procedure. The various monosaccharide methyl ethers produced by the methylation are separated by gas–liquid chromatography.

Detailed statements about polysaccharide structure and function are limited by the statistical nature of some measurements (e.g., branching frequency), the biological variability of parameters such as size and molecular weight, and incomplete information about associative interactions in living things.

Protein

Protein is a highly complex substance that is present in all living organisms. Proteins are of great nutritional value and are directly involved in the chemical processes essential for life.

A protein molecule is very large compared with molecules of sugar or salt and consists of many amino acids joined together to form long chains, much as beads are arranged on a string. There are about 20 different amino acids that occur naturally in proteins. Proteins of similar function have similar amino acid composition and sequence. Although it is not yet possible to explain all of the functions of a protein from its amino acid sequence, established correlations between structure and function can be attributed to the properties of the amino acids that compose proteins.

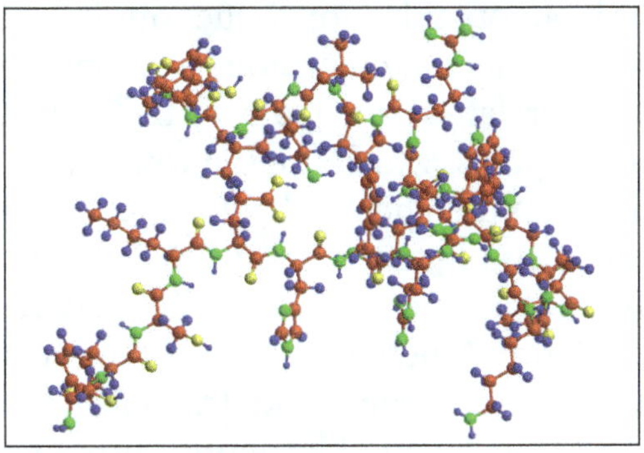

Peptide: The molecular structure of a peptide (a small protein) consists of a sequence of amino acids

Plants can synthesize all of the amino acids; animals cannot, even though all of them are essential for life. Plants can grow in a medium containing inorganic nutrients that provide nitrogen, potassium, and other substances essential for growth. They utilize the carbon dioxide in the air during the process of photosynthesis to form organic compounds such as carbohydrates. Animals, however, must obtain organic nutrients from outside sources. Because the protein content of most plants is low, very large amounts of plant material are required by animals, such as ruminants (e.g., cows), that eat only plant material to meet their amino acid requirements. Nonruminant animals, including humans, obtain proteins principally from animals and their products-e.g., meat, milk, and eggs. The seeds of legumes are increasingly being used to prepare inexpensive protein-rich food.

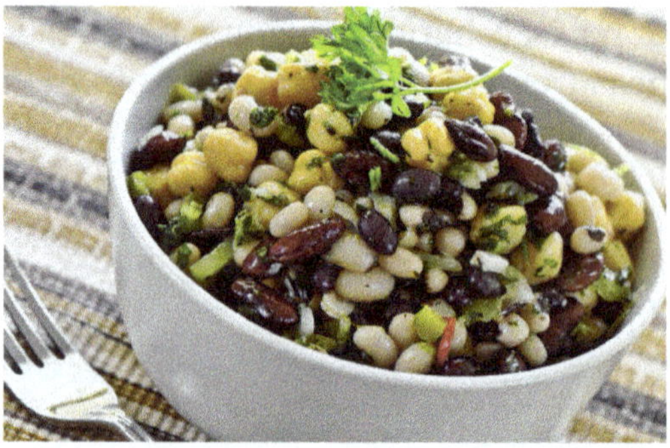

Legume (amino acid) Legumes—such as beans, lentils, and peas—are high in protein and contain many essential amino acids

The protein content of animal organs is usually much higher than that of the blood plasma. Muscles, for example, contain about 30 percent protein, the liver 20 to 30 percent, and red blood cells 30 percent. Higher percentages of protein are found in hair, bones, and other organs and tissues with a low water content. The quantity of free amino acids and peptides in animals is much smaller than the amount of protein; protein molecules are produced in cells by the stepwise alignment of amino acids and are released into the body fluids only after synthesis is complete.

The high protein content of some organs does not mean that the importance of proteins is related to their amount in an organism or tissue; on the contrary, some of the most important proteins, such as enzymes and hormones, occur in extremely small amounts. The importance of proteins is related principally to their function. All enzymes identified thus far are proteins. Enzymes, which are the catalysts of all metabolic reactions, enable an organism to build up the chemical substances necessary for life—proteins, nucleic acids, carbohydrates, and lipids—to convert them into other substances, and to degrade them. Life without enzymes is not possible. There are several protein hormones with important regulatory functions. In all vertebrates, the respiratory protein hemoglobin acts as oxygen carrier in the blood, transporting oxygen from the lung to body organs and tissues. A large group of structural proteins maintains and protects the structure of the animal body.

In figure, each chain is attached to a heme group composed of porphyrin (an organic ringlike compound) attached to an iron atom. These iron-porphyrin complexes coordinate oxygen molecules reversibly, an ability directly related to the role of hemoglobin in oxygen transport in the blood.

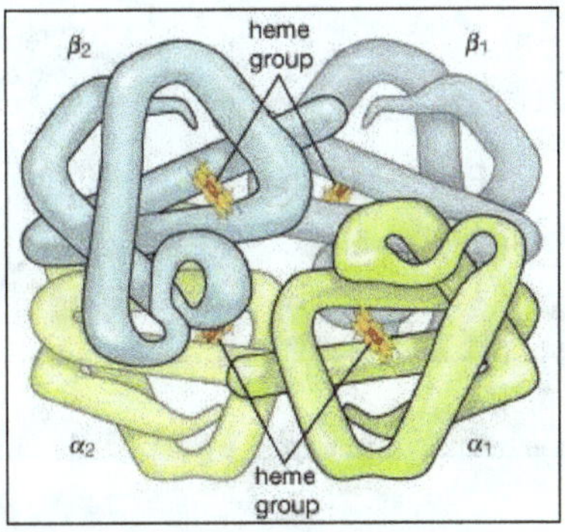

Hemoglobin is a protein made up of four polypeptide chains (α_1, α_2, β_1, and β_2)

General Structure and Properties of Proteins

The Amino Acid Composition of Proteins

The common property of all proteins is that they consist of long chains of α-amino (alpha amino) acids. The general structure of α-amino acids is shown in . The α-amino acids are so called because the α-carbon atom in the molecule carries an amino group ($-NH_2$); the α-carbon atom also carries a carboxyl group (-COOH).

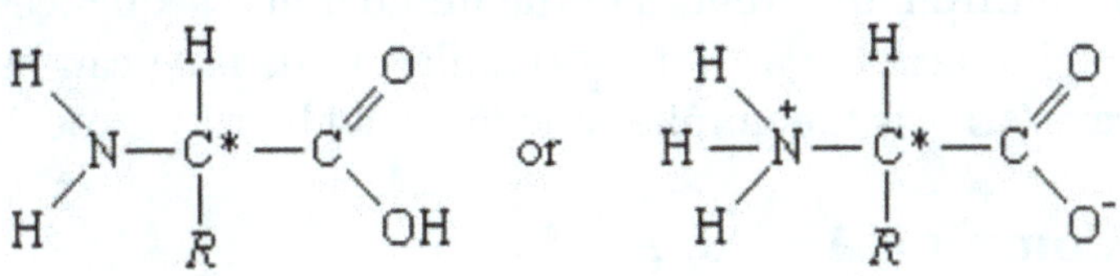

In acidic solutions, when the pH is less than 4, the -COO groups combine with hydrogen ions (H^+) and are thus converted into the uncharged form (-COOH). In alkaline solutions, at pH above 9, the ammonium groups ($-NH^+{}_3$) lose a hydrogen ion and are converted into amino groups ($-NH_2$). In the pH range between 4 and 8, amino acids carry both a positive and a negative charge and therefore do not migrate in an electrical field. Such structures have been designated as dipolar ions, or zwitterions (i.e., hybrid ions).

Although more than 100 amino acids occur in nature, particularly in plants, only 20 types are commonly found in most proteins. In protein molecules the α-amino acids are linked to each other by peptide bonds between the amino group of one amino acid and the carboxyl group of its neighbour.

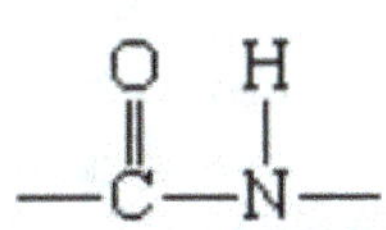

The condensation (joining) of three amino acids yields the tripeptide.

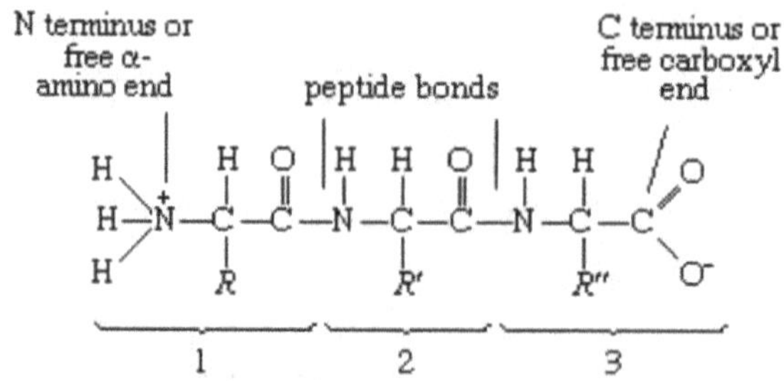

three amino acids joined by peptide bonds

It is customary to write the structure of peptides in such a way that the free α-amino group (also called the N terminus of the peptide) is at the left side and the free carboxyl group (the C terminus) at the right side. Proteins are macromolecular polypeptides—i.e., very large molecules (macromolecules) composed of many peptide-bonded amino acids. Most of the common ones contain more than 100 amino acids linked to each other in a long peptide chain. The average molecular weight (based on the weight of a hydrogen atom as 1) of each amino acid is approximately 100 to 125; thus, the molecular weights of proteins are usually in the range of 10,000 to 100,000 daltons (one dalton is the weight of one hydrogen atom). The species-specificity and organ-specificity of proteins result from differences in the number and sequences of amino acids. Twenty different amino acids in a chain 100 amino acids long can be arranged in far more than 10^{100} ways (10^{100} is the number one followed by 100 zeroes).

Structures of Common Amino Acids

The amino acids present in proteins differ from each other in the structure of their side (R) chains. The simplest amino acid is glycine, in which R is a hydrogen atom. In a number of amino acids, R represents straight or branched carbon chains. One of these amino acids is alanine, in which R is the methyl group ($-CH_3$). Valine, leucine, and isoleucine, with longer R groups, complete the alkyl side-chain series. The alkyl side chains (R groups) of these amino acids are nonpolar; this means that they have no affinity for water but some affinity for each other. Although plants can form all of the alkyl amino acids, animals can synthesize only alanine and glycine; thus valine, leucine, and isoleucine must be supplied in the diet.

Two amino acids, each containing three carbon atoms, are derived from alanine; they are serine and cysteine. Serine contains an alcohol group ($-CH_2OH$) instead of the methyl group of alanine, and cysteine contains a mercapto group ($-CH_2SH$). Animals can synthesize serine but not cysteine or cystine. Cysteine occurs in proteins predominantly in its oxidized form (oxidation in this sense meaning the removal of hydrogen atoms), called cystine. Cystine consists of two cysteine molecules linked by the disulfide bond (-S-S-) that results when a hydrogen atom is removed from the mercapto group of each of the cysteines. Disulfide bonds are important in protein structure because they allow the linkage of two different parts of a protein molecule to-and thus the formation of loops in-the otherwise straight chains. Some proteins contain small amounts of cysteine with free sulfhydryl (-SH) groups.

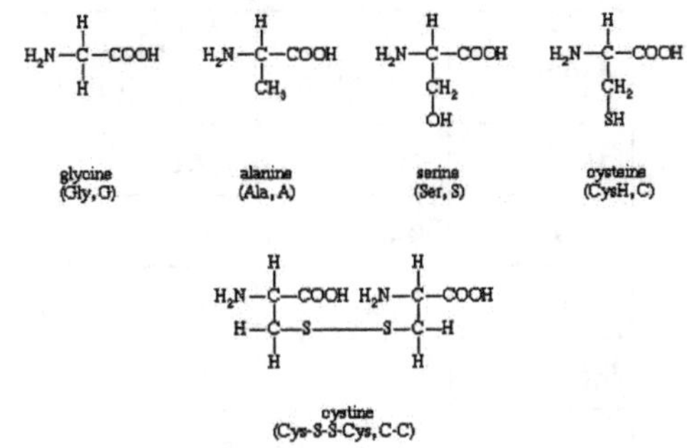

Four amino acids, each consisting of four carbon atoms, occur in proteins; they are aspartic acid, asparagine, threonine, and methionine. Aspartic acid and asparagine, which occur in large amounts, can be synthesized by animals. Threonine and methionine cannot be synthesized and thus are essential amino acids; i.e., they must be supplied in the diet. Most proteins contain only small amounts of methionine.

Proteins also contain an amino acid with five carbon atoms (glutamic acid) and a secondary amine (in proline), which is a structure with the amino group ($-NH_2$) bonded to the alkyl side chain, forming a ring. Glutamic acid and aspartic acid are dicarboxylic acids; that is, they have two carboxyl groups (-COOH).

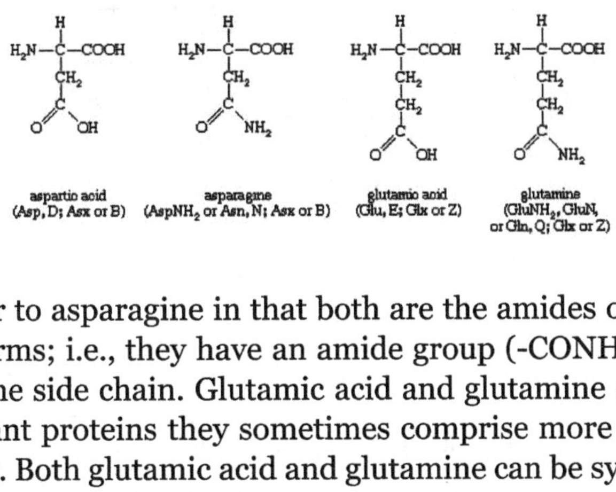

Glutamine is similar to asparagine in that both are the amides of their corresponding dicarboxylic acid forms; i.e., they have an amide group ($-CONH_2$) in place of the carboxyl (-COOH) of the side chain. Glutamic acid and glutamine are abundant in most proteins; e.g., in plant proteins they sometimes comprise more than one-third of the amino acids present. Both glutamic acid and glutamine can be synthesized by animals.

Amino acid content of some proteins*						
Amino Acid	Protein					
	Alpha-casein	Gliadin	Edestin	Collagen (oxhide)	Keratin (wool)	Myosin
lysine	60.9	4.45	19.9	27.4	6.2	85
histidine	18.7	11.7	18.6	4.5	19.7	15

Amino acid content of some proteins*						
Amino Acid	Protein					
	Alpha-casein	Gliadin	Edestin	Collagen (oxhide)	Keratin (wool)	Myosin
arginine	24.7	15.7	99.2	47.1	56.9	41
aspartic acid**	63.1	10.1	99.4	51.9	51.5	85
threonine	41.2	17.6	31.2	19.3	55.9	41
serine	63.1	46.7	55.7	41.0	79.5	41
glutamic acid**	153.1	311.0	144.9	76.2	99.0	155
proline	71.3	117.8	32.9	125.2	58.3	22
glycine	37.3	—	68.0	354.6	78.0	39
alanine	41.5	23.9	57.7	115.7	43.8	78
half-cystine	3.6	21.3	10.9	0.0	105.0	86
valine	53.8	22.7	54.6	21.4	46.6	42
methionine	16.8	11.3	16.4	6.5	4.0	22
isoleucine	48.8	90.8***	41.9	14.5	29.0	42
leucine	60.3		60.0	28.2	59.9	79
tyrosine	44.7	17.7	26.9	5.5	28.7	18
phenylalanine	27.9	39.0	38.4	13.9	22.4	27
tryptophan	7.8	3.2	6.6	0.0	9.6	—
hydroxyproline	0.0	0.0	0.0	97.5	12.2	—
hydroxylysine	—	—	—	8.0	1.2	—
total	839	765	883	1,058	863	832
average residual weight	119	131	113	95	117	120
*Number of gram molecules of amino acid per 100,000 grams of protein.						
**The values for aspartic acid and glutamic acid include asparagine and glutamine, respectively.						
***Isoleucine plus leucine.						

The amino acids proline and hydroxyproline occur in large amounts in collagen, the protein of the connective tissue of animals. Proline and hydroxyproline lack free amino (-NH_2) groups because the amino group is enclosed in a ring structure with the side chain; they thus cannot exist in a zwitterion form. Although the nitrogen-containing group (>NH) of these amino acids can form a peptide bond with the carboxyl group of another amino acid, the bond so formed gives rise to a kink in the peptide chain; i.e., the ring structure alters the regular bond angle of normal peptide bonds.

Proteins usually are almost neutral molecules; that is, they have neither acidic nor basic properties. This means that the acidic carboxyl (-COO^-) groups of aspartic and glutamic acid are about equal in number to the amino acids with basic side chains. Three such basic amino acids, each containing six carbon atoms, occur in proteins. The one with the simplest structure, lysine, is synthesized by plants but not by animals. Even some plants have a low lysine content. Arginine is found in all proteins; it occurs in particularly high amounts in the strongly basic protamines (simple proteins composed of relatively few amino acids) of fish sperm. The third basic amino acid is histidine. Both arginine and histidine can be synthesized by animals. Histidine is a weaker base than either lysine or arginine. The imidazole ring, a five-membered ring structure containing two nitrogen atoms in the side chain of histidine, acts as a buffer (i.e., a stabilizer of hydrogen ion concentration) by binding hydrogen ions (H^+) to the nitrogen atoms of the imidazole ring.

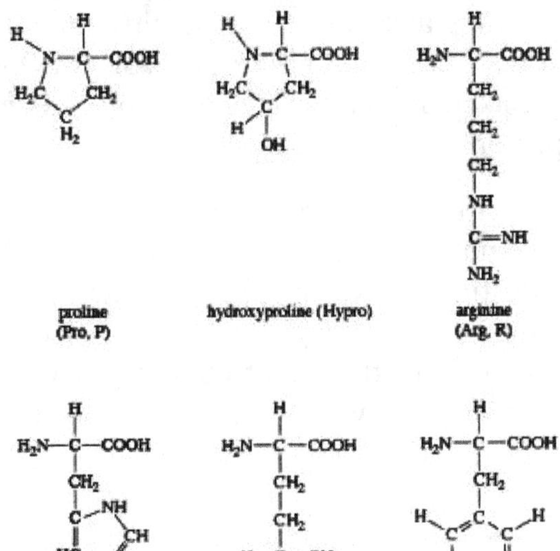

proline (Pro, P) — hydroxyproline (Hypro) — arginine (Arg, R)

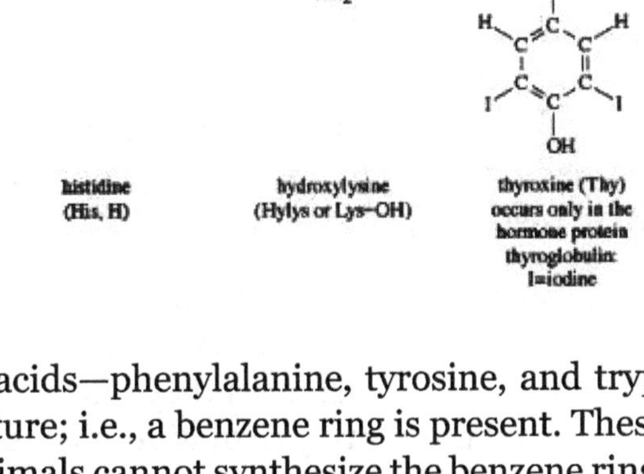

histidine (His, H) — hydroxylysine (Hylys or Lys–OH) — thyroxine (Thy) occurs only in the hormone protein thyroglobulin I=iodine

The remaining amino acids—phenylalanine, tyrosine, and tryptophan—have in common an aromatic structure; i.e., a benzene ring is present. These three amino acids are essential, and, while animals cannot synthesize the benzene ring itself, they can convert phenylalanine to tyrosine.

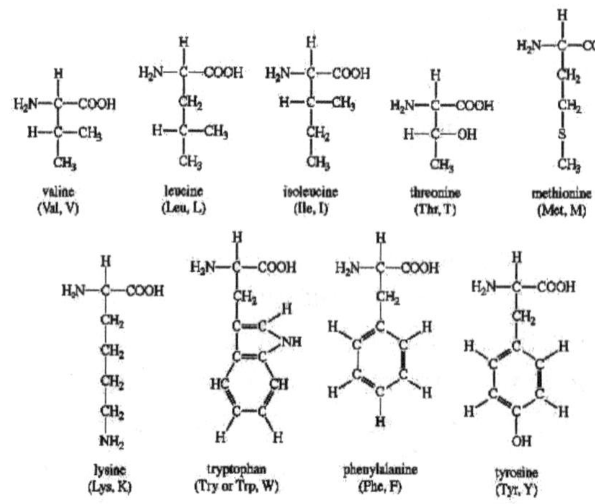

Because these amino acids contain benzene rings, they can absorb ultraviolet light at wavelengths between 270 and 290 nanometres (nm; 1 nanometre = 10^{-9} metre = 10 angstrom units). Phenylalanine absorbs very little ultraviolet light; tyrosine and tryptophan, however, absorb it strongly and are responsible for the absorption band most proteins exhibit at 280–290 nanometres. This absorption is often used to determine the quantity of protein present in protein samples.

Most proteins contain only the amino acids described above; however, other amino acids occur in proteins in small amounts. For example, the collagen found in connective tissue contains, in addition to hydroxyproline, small amounts of hydroxylysine. Other proteins contain some monomethyl-, dimethyl-, or trimethyllysine-i.e., lysine derivatives containing one, two, or three methyl groups ($-CH_3$). The amount of these unusual amino acids in proteins, however, rarely exceeds 1 or 2 percent of the total amino acids.

Physicochemical Properties of the Amino Acids

The physicochemical properties of a protein are determined by the analogous properties of the amino acids in it.

The α-carbon atom of all amino acids, with the exception of glycine, is asymmetric; this means that four different chemical entities (atoms or groups of atoms) are attached to it. As a result, each of the amino acids, except glycine, can exist in two different spatial, or geometric, arrangements (i.e., isomers), which are mirror images akin to right and left hands.

These isomers exhibit the property of optical rotation. Optical rotation is the rotation of the plane of polarized light, which is composed of light waves that vibrate in one plane, or direction, only. Solutions of substances that rotate the plane of polarization are said to be optically active, and the degree of rotation is called the optical rotation of the solution. The direction in which the light is rotated is generally designed as plus, or d, for dextrorotatory (to the right), or as minus, or l, for levorotatory (to the left). Some amino acids are dextrorotatory, others are levorotatory. With the exception of a few small proteins (peptides) that occur in bacteria, the amino acids that occur in proteins are L-amino acids.

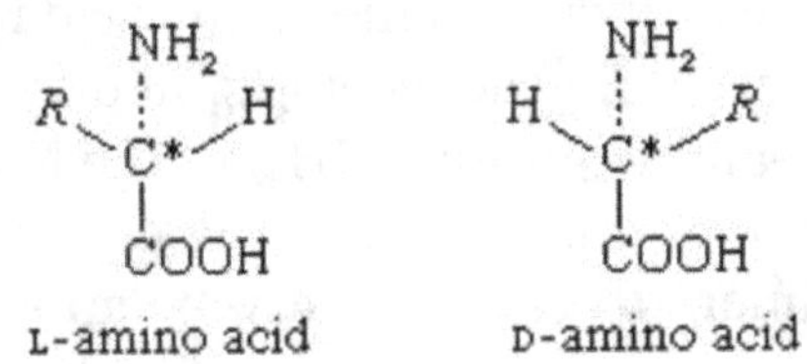

In bacteria, D-alanine and some other D-amino acids have been found as components of gramicidin and bacitracin. These peptides are toxic to other bacteria and are used in medicine as antibiotics. The D-alanine has also been found in some peptides of bacterial membranes.

In contrast to most organic acids and amines, the amino acids are insoluble in organic solvents. In aqueous solutions they are dipolar ions (zwitterions, or hybrid ions) that react with strong acids or bases in a way that leads to the neutralization of the negatively or positively charged ends, respectively. Because of their reactions with strong acids and strong bases, the amino acids act as buffers-stabilizers of hydrogen ion (H^+) or hydroxide ion (OH^-) concentrations. In fact, glycine is frequently used as a buffer in the pH range from 1 to 3 (acid solutions) and from 9 to 12 (basic solutions). In acid solutions, glycine has a positive charge and therefore migrates to the cathode (negative electrode of a direct-current electrical circuit with terminals in the solution). Its charge, however, is negative in alkaline solutions, in which it migrates to the anode (positive electrode). At pH 6.1 glycine does not migrate, because each molecule has one positive and one negative charge. The pH at which an amino acid does not migrate in an electrical field is called the isoelectric point. Most of the monoamino acids (i.e., those with only one amino group) have isoelectric points similar to that of glycine. The isoelectric points of aspartic and glutamic acids, however, are close to pH 3, and those of histidine, lysine, and arginine are at pH 7.6, 9.7, and 10.8, respectively.

Amino Acid Sequence in Protein Molecules

Since each protein molecule consists of a long chain of amino acid residues, linked to each other by peptide bonds, the hydrolytic cleavage of all peptide bonds is a prerequisite for the quantitative determination of the amino acid residues. Hydrolysis is most frequently accomplished by boiling the protein with concentrated hydrochloric acid. The quantitative determination of the amino acids is based on the discovery that amino acids can be separated from each other by chromatography on filter paper and made visible by spraying the paper with ninhydrin. The amino acids of the protein hydrolysate are separated from each other by passing the hydrolysate through a column of adsorbents, which adsorb the amino acids with different affinities and, on washing the column with buffer solutions, release them in a definite order. The amount of each of the amino acids can be determined by the intensity of the colour reaction with ninhydrin.

To obtain information about the sequence of the amino acid residues in the protein, the protein is degraded stepwise, one amino acid being split off in each step. This is accomplished by coupling the free α-amino group ($-NH_2$) of the N-terminal amino acid with phenyl isothiocyanate; subsequent mild hydrolysis does not affect the peptide bonds. The procedure, called the Edman degradation, can be applied repeatedly; it thus reveals the sequence of the amino acids in the peptide chain.

Unavoidable small losses that occur during each step make it impossible to determine the sequence of more than about 30 to 50 amino acids by this procedure. For this reason the protein is usually first hydrolyzed by exposure to the enzyme trypsin, which cleaves only peptide bonds formed by the carboxyl groups of lysine and arginine.

Levels of Structural Organization in Proteins

Primary Structure

Analytical and synthetic procedures reveal only the primary structure of the proteins-that is, the amino acid sequence of the peptide chains. They do not reveal information about the conformation (arrangement in space) of the peptide chain-that is, whether the peptide chain is present as a long straight thread or is irregularly coiled and folded into a globule. The configuration, or conformation, of a protein is determined by mutual attraction or repulsion of polar or nonpolar groups in the side chains (R groups) of the amino acids. The former have positive or negative charges in their side chains; the latter repel water but attract each other. Some parts of a peptide chain containing 100 to 200 amino acids may form a loop, or helix; others may be straight or form irregular coils.

The primary structure of a protein is determined by its amino acid sequence without any regard for the arrangement of the peptide chain in space. The secondary structure is determined by the spatial arrangement of the main peptide chain without any regard for the conformation of side chains or other segments of the main chain. The tertiary structure is determined by both the side chains and other adjacent segments of the main chain, without regard for neighbouring peptide chains. Finally, the term quaternary structure is used for the arrangement of identical or different subunits of a large protein in which each subunit is a separate peptide chain.

Secondary Structure

The nitrogen and carbon atoms of a peptide chain cannot lie on a straight line, because of the magnitude of the bond angles between adjacent atoms of the chain; the bond angle is about 110°. Each of the nitrogen and carbon atoms can rotate to a certain extent, however, so that the chain has a limited flexibility. Because all of the amino acids, except glycine, are asymmetric L-amino acids, the peptide chain tends to assume an asymmetric helical shape; some of the fibrous proteins consist of elongated helices around a straight screw axis. Such structural features result from properties common to all peptide chains. The product of their effects is the secondary structure of the protein.

Tertiary Structure

The tertiary structure is the product of the interaction between the side chains (R) of the amino acids composing the protein. Some of them contain positively or negatively charged groups, others are polar, and still others are nonpolar. The number of carbon atoms in the side chain varies from zero in glycine to nine in tryptophan. Positively and negatively charged side chains have the tendency to attract each other; side chains with identical charges repel each other. The bonds formed by the forces between the negatively charged side chains of aspartic or glutamic acid on the one hand, and the positively charged side chains of lysine or arginine on the other hand, are called salt bridges. Mutual attraction of adjacent peptide chains also results from the formation of numerous hydrogen bonds.

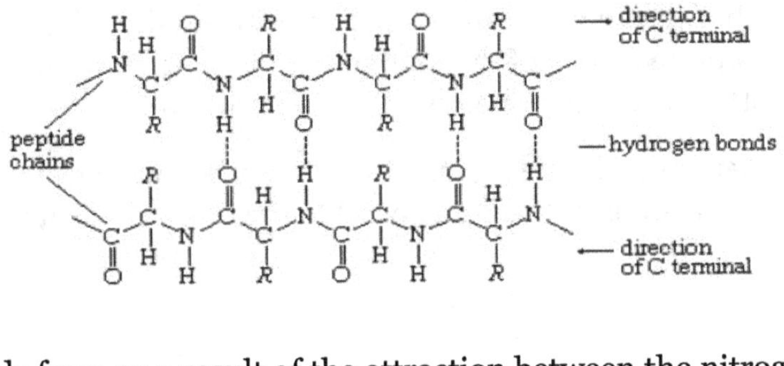

Hydrogen bonds form as a result of the attraction between the nitrogen-bound hydrogen atom (the imide hydrogen) and the unshared pair of electrons of the oxygen atom in the double bonded carbon–oxygen group (the carbonyl group). The result is a slight displacement of the imide hydrogen toward the oxygen atom of the carbonyl group. Although the hydrogen bond is much weaker than a covalent bond (i.e., the type of bond between two carbon atoms, which equally share the pair of bonding electrons between them), the large number of imide and carbonyl groups in peptide chains results in the formation of numerous hydrogen bonds. Another type of attraction is that between nonpolar side chains of valine, leucine, isoleucine, and phenylalanine; the attraction results in the displacement of water molecules and is called hydrophobic interaction.

In proteins rich in cystine, the conformation of the peptide chain is determined to a considerable extent by the disulfide bonds (-S-S-) of cystine. The halves of cystine may be located in different parts of the peptide chain and thus may form a loop closed by the disulfide bond.

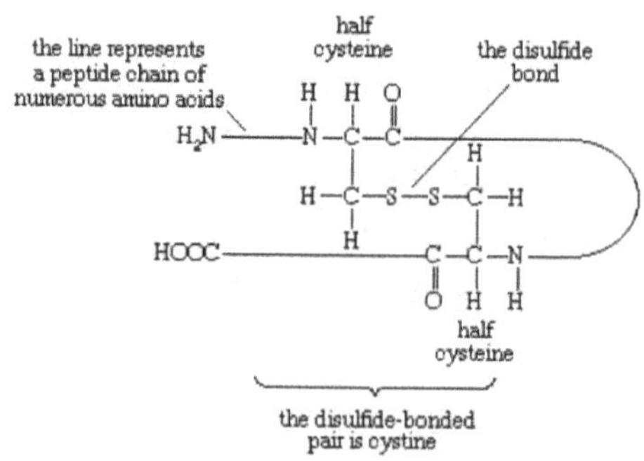

If the disulfide bond is reduced (i.e., hydrogen is added) to two sulfhydryl (-SH) groups, the tertiary structure of the protein undergoes a drastic change—closed loops are broken and adjacent disulfide-bonded peptide chains separate.

Quaternary Structure

The nature of the quaternary structure is demonstrated by the structure of hemoglobin. Each molecule of human hemoglobin consists of four peptide chains, two α-chains and two β-chains; i.e., it is a tetramer. The four subunits are linked to each other by hydrogen bonds and hydrophobic interaction. Because the four subunits are so closely linked, the hemoglobin tetramer is called a molecule, even though no covalent bonds occur between the peptide chains of the four subunits. In other proteins, the subunits are bound to each other by covalent bonds (disulfide bridges).

The amino acid sequence of porcine proinsulin is shown below. The arrows indicate the direction from the N terminus of the β-chain (B) to the C terminus of the α-chain (A).

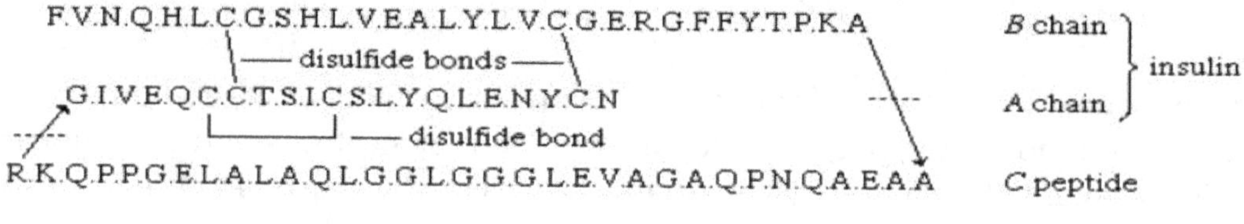

The Isolation and Determination of Proteins

Animal material usually contains large amounts of protein and lipids and small amounts of carbohydrate; in plants, the bulk of the dry matter is usually carbohydrate. If it is necessary to determine the amount of protein in a mixture of animal foodstuffs, a sample is converted to ammonium salts by boiling with sulfuric acid and a suitable inorganic catalyst, such as copper sulfate (Kjeldahl method). The method is based on the assumption that proteins contain 16 percent nitrogen, and that nonprotein nitrogen is present in very small amounts. The assumption is justified for most tissues from higher animals but not for insects and crustaceans, in which a considerable portion of the body nitrogen is present in the form of chitin, a carbohydrate. Large amounts of nonprotein nitrogen are also found in the sap of many plants. In such cases, the precise quantitative analyses are made after the proteins have been separated from other biological compounds.

Proteins are sensitive to heat, acids, bases, organic solvents, and radiation exposure; for this reason, the chemical methods employed to purify organic compounds cannot be applied to proteins. Salts and molecules of small size are removed from protein solutions by dialysis—i.e., by placing the solution into a sac of semipermeable material, such as cellulose or acetylcellulose, which will allow small molecules to pass through but not large protein molecules, and immersing the sac in water or a salt solution. Small molecules can also be removed either by passing the protein solution through a column of resin that adsorbs only the protein or by gel filtration. In gel filtration, the large protein molecules pass through the column, and the small molecules are adsorbed to the gel.

Groups of proteins are separated from each other by salting out-i.e., the stepwise addition of sodium sulfate or ammonium sulfate to a protein solution. Some proteins, called globulins, become insoluble and precipitate when the solution is half-saturated with ammonium sulfate or when its sodium sulfate content exceeds about 12 percent. Other proteins, the albumins, can be precipitated from the supernatant solution (i.e., the solution remaining after a precipitation has taken place) by saturation with ammonium sulfate. Water-soluble proteins can be obtained in a dry state by freeze-drying (lyophilization), in which the protein solution is deep-frozen by lowering the temperature below −15 °C (5 °F) and removing the water; the protein is obtained as a dry powder.

Most proteins are insoluble in boiling water and are denatured by it-i.e., irreversibly converted into an insoluble material. Heat denaturation cannot be used with connective tissue because the principal structural protein, collagen, is converted by boiling water into water-soluble gelatin.

Fractionation (separation into components) of a mixture of proteins of different molecular weight can be accomplished by gel filtration. The size of the proteins retained by the gel depends upon the properties of the gel. The proteins retained in the gel are removed from the column by solutions of a suitable concentration of salts and hydrogen ions.

Many proteins were originally obtained in crystalline form, but crystallinity is not proof of purity; many crystalline protein preparations contain other substances. Various tests are used to determine whether a protein preparation contains only one protein. The purity of a protein solution can be determined by such techniques as chromatography and gel filtration. In addition, a solution of pure protein will yield one peak when spun in a centrifuge at very high speeds (ultracentrifugation) and will migrate as a single band in electrophoresis (migration of the protein in an electrical field). After these methods and others (such as amino acid analysis) indicate that the protein solution is pure, it can be considered so. Because chromatography, ultracentrifugation, and electrophoresis cannot be applied to insoluble proteins, little is known about them; they may be mixtures of many similar proteins.

Very small (microheterogeneous) differences in some of the apparently pure proteins are known to occur. They are differences in the amino acid composition of otherwise identical proteins and are transmitted from generation to generation; i.e., they are genetically determined. For example, some humans have two hemoglobins, hemoglobin A and hemoglobin S, which differ in one amino acid at a specific site in the molecule. In hemoglobin A the site is occupied by glutamic acid and in hemoglobin S by valine. Refinement of the techniques of protein analysis has resulted in the discovery of other instances of microheterogeneity.

The quantity of a pure protein can be determined by weighing or by measuring the ultraviolet absorbancy at 280 nanometres. The absorbency at 280 nanometres depends on the content of tyrosine and tryptophan in the protein. Sometimes the slightly less sensitive biuret reaction, a purple colour given by alkaline protein solutions upon the addition of copper sulfate, is used; its intensity depends only on the number of peptide bonds per gram, which is similar in all proteins.

Physicochemical Properties of Proteins

The Molecular Weight of Proteins

The molecular weight of proteins cannot be determined by the methods of classical chemistry (e.g., freezing-point depression), because they require solutions of a higher concentration of protein than can be prepared.

If a protein contains only one molecule of one of the amino acids or one atom of iron, copper, or another element, the minimum molecular weight of the protein or a subunit can be calculated; for example, the protein myoglobin contains 0.34 gram of iron in 100 grams of protein. The atomic weight of iron is 56; thus the minimum molecular weight of myoglobin is $(56 \times 100)/0.34$ = about 16,500. Direct measurements of the molecular weight of myoglobin yield the same value. The molecular weight of hemoglobin, however, which also contains 0.34 percent iron, has been found to be 66,000 or $4 \times 16{,}500$; thus hemoglobin contains four atoms of iron.

The method most frequently used to determine the molecular weight of proteins is ultracentrifugation-i.e., spinning in a centrifuge at velocities up to about 60,000 revolutions per minute. Centrifugal forces of more than 200,000 times the gravitational force on the surface of Earth are achieved at such velocities. The first ultracentrifuges, built in 1920, were used to determine the molecular weight of proteins. The molecular weights of a large number of proteins have been determined. Most consist of several subunits, the molecular weight of which is usually less than 100,000 and frequently ranges from 20,000 to 30,000. Proteins of very high molecular weights are found among hemocyanins, the copper-containing respiratory proteins of invertebrates; some range as high as several million. Although there is no definite lower limit for the molecular weight of proteins, short amino acid sequences are usually called peptides.

The Shape of Protein Molecules

In the technique of X-ray diffraction, the X-rays are allowed to strike a protein crystal. The X-rays, diffracted (bent) by the crystal, impinge on a photographic plate, forming a pattern of spots. This method reveals that peptide chains can assume very complicated, apparently irregular shapes. Two extremes in shape include the closely folded structure of the globular proteins and the elongated, unidimensional structure of the threadlike fibrous proteins; both were recognized many years before the technique of X-ray diffraction was developed. Solutions of fibrous proteins are extremely viscous (i.e., sticky); those of the globular proteins have low viscosity (i.e., they flow easily). A 5 percent solution of a globular protein-ovalbumin, for example-easily flows through a narrow glass tube; a 5 percent solution of gelatin, a fibrous protein, however, does not flow through the tube, because it is liquid only at high temperatures and solidifies at room temperature. Even solutions containing only 1 or 2 percent of gelatin are highly viscous and flow through a narrow tube either very slowly or only under pressure.

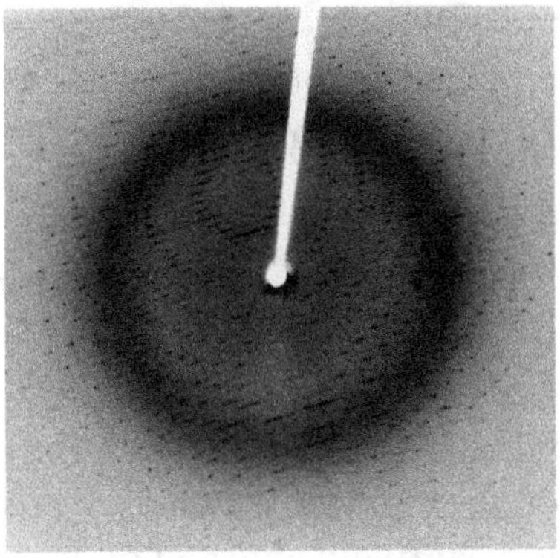

X-ray diffraction: X-ray diffraction pattern of a crystallized enzyme

The elongated peptide chains of the fibrous proteins can be imagined to become entangled not only mechanically but also by mutual attraction of their side chains, and in this way they incorporate large amounts of water. Most of the hydrophilic (water-attracting) groups of the globular proteins, however, lie on the surface of the molecules, and, as a result, globular proteins incorporate only a few water molecules. If a solution of a fibrous protein flows through a narrow tube, the elongated molecules become oriented parallel to the direction of the flow, and the solution thus becomes birefringent like a crystal; i.e., it splits a light ray into two components that travel at different velocities and are polarized at right angles to each other. Globular proteins do not show this phenomenon, which is called flow birefringence. Solutions of myosin, the contractile protein of muscles, show very high flow birefringence; other proteins with very high flow birefringence include solutions of fibrinogen, the clotting material of blood plasma, and solutions of tobacco mosaic virus. The gamma-globulins of the blood plasma show low flow birefringence, and none can be observed in solutions of serum albumin and ovalbumin.

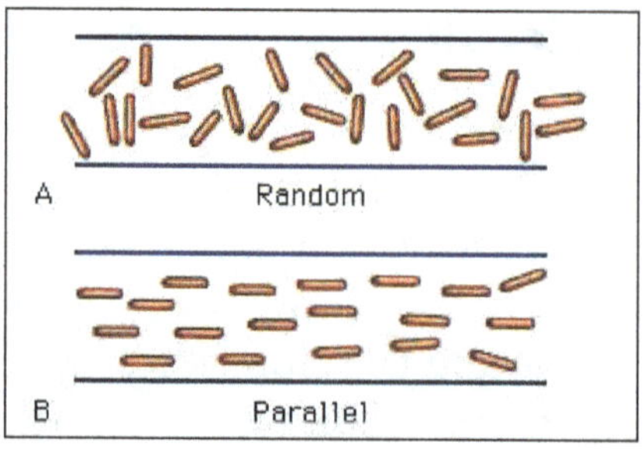

Flow birefringence: Orientation of elongated, rodlike macromolecules (A) in resting solution, or (B) during flow through a horizontal tube

Hydration of Proteins

When dry proteins are exposed to air of high water content, they rapidly bind water up to a maximum quantity, which differs for different proteins; usually it is 10 to 20 percent of the weight of the protein. The hydrophilic groups of a protein are chiefly the positively charged groups in the side chains of lysine and arginine and the negatively charged groups of aspartic and glutamic acid. Hydration (i.e., the binding of water) may also occur at the hydroxyl (-OH) groups of serine and threonine or at the amide (-$CONH_2$) groups of asparagine and glutamine.

The binding of water molecules to either charged or polar (partly charged) groups is explained by the dipolar structure of the water molecule; that is, the two positively charged hydrogen atoms form an angle of about 105°, with the negatively charged oxygen atom at the apex. The centre of the positive charges is located between the two hydrogen atoms; the centre of the negative charge of the oxygen atom is at the apex of the angle. The negative pole of the dipolar water molecule binds to positively charged groups; the positive pole binds negatively charged ones. The negative pole of the water molecule also binds to the hydroxyl and amino groups of the protein.

The water of hydration is essential to the structure of protein crystals; when they are completely dehydrated, the crystalline structure disintegrates. In some proteins this process is accompanied by denaturation and loss of the biological function.

In aqueous solutions, proteins bind some of the water molecules very firmly; others are either very loosely bound or form islands of water molecules between loops of folded peptide chains. Because the water molecules in such an island are thought to be oriented as in ice, which is crystalline water, the islands of water in proteins are called icebergs. Water molecules may also form bridges between the carbonyl and imino groups of adjacent peptide chains, resulting in structures similar to those of the pleated sheet but with a water molecule in the position of the hydrogen bonds of that configuration. The extent of hydration of protein molecules in aqueous solutions is important, because some of the methods used to determine the molecular weight of proteins yield the molecular weight of the hydrated protein. The amount of water bound to one gram of a globular protein in solution varies from 0.2 to 0.5 gram. Much larger amounts of water are mechanically immobilized between the elongated peptide chains of fibrous proteins; for example, one gram of gelatin can immobilize at room temperature 25 to 30 grams of water.

Hydration of proteins is necessary for their solubility in water. If the water of hydration of a protein dissolved in water is reduced by the addition of a salt such as ammonium sulfate, the protein is no longer soluble and is salted out, or precipitated. The salting-out process is reversible because the protein is not denatured (i.e., irreversibly converted to an insoluble material) by the addition of such salts as sodium chloride, sodium sulfate, or ammonium sulfate. Some globulins, called euglobulins, are insoluble in water in the absence of salts; their insolubility is attributed to the mutual interaction of polar groups on the surface of adjacent molecules, a process that results in the formation of large aggregates of molecules. Addition of small amounts of salt causes the euglobulins to become soluble. This process, called salting in, results from a combination between anions (negatively charged ions) and cations (positively charged ions) of the salt and positively and negatively charged side chains of the euglobulins. The combination prevents the aggregation of euglobulin molecules by preventing the formation of salt bridges between them. The addition of more sodium or ammonium sulfate causes the euglobulins to salt out again and to precipitate.

Electrochemistry of Proteins

Because the α-amino group and α-carboxyl group of amino acids are converted into peptide bonds in the protein molecule, there is only one α-amino group (at the N terminus) and one α-carboxyl group (at the C terminus) in a given protein molecule. The electrochemical character of a protein is affected very little by these two groups. Of importance, however, are the numerous positively charged ammonium groups ($-NH_3^+$) of lysine and arginine and the negatively charged carboxyl groups ($-COO^-$) of aspartic acid and glutamic acid. In most proteins, the number of positively and negatively charged groups varies from 10 to 20 per 100 amino acids.

Electrometric Titration

When measured volumes of hydrochloric acid are added to a solution of protein in salt-free water, the pH decreases in proportion to the amount of hydrogen ions added until it is about 4. Further addition of acid causes much less decrease in pH because the protein acts as a buffer at pH values of 3 to 4. The reaction that takes place in this pH range is the protonation of the carboxyl group-i.e., the conversion of $-COO^-$ into -COOH. Electrometric titration of an isoelectric protein with potassium hydroxide causes a very slow increase in pH and a weak buffering action of the protein at pH 7; a very strong buffering action occurs in the pH range from 9 to 10. The buffering action at pH 7, which is caused by loss of protons (positively charged hydrogen) from the imidazolium groups (i.e., the five-member ring structure in the side chain) of histidine, is weak because the histidine content of proteins is usually low. The much stronger buffering action at pH values from 9 to 10 is caused by the loss of protons from the hydroxyl group of tyrosine and from the ammonium groups of lysine. Finally, protons are lost from the guanidinium groups (i.e., the nitrogen-containing terminal portion of the arginine side chains) of arginine at pH 12. Electrometric titrations of proteins yield similar curves. Electrometric titration makes possible the determination of the approximate number of carboxyl groups, ammonium groups, histidines, and tyrosines per molecule of protein.

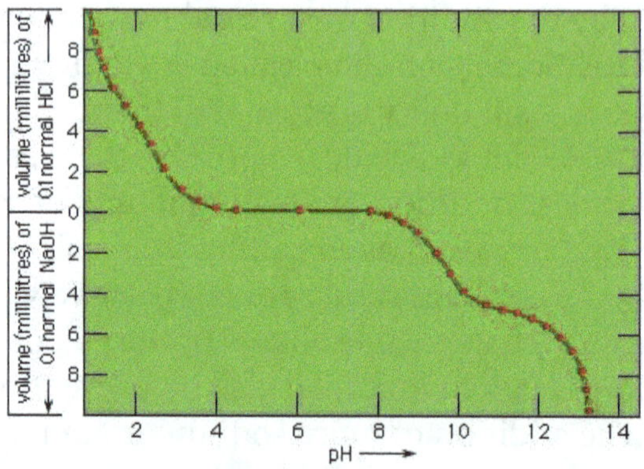

Electrometric titration of glycine

Electrophoresis

The positively and negatively charged side chains of proteins cause them to behave like amino acids in an electrical field; that is, they migrate during electrophoresis at low pH values to the cathode (negative terminal) and at high pH values to the anode (positive terminal). The isoelectric point, the pH value at which the protein molecule does not migrate, is in the range of pH 5 to 7 for many proteins. Proteins such as lysozyme, cytochrome c, histone, and others rich in lysine and arginine, however, have isoelectric points in the pH range between 8 and 10. The isoelectric point of pepsin, which contains very few basic amino acids, is close to 1.

Number of amino acids per protein molecule							
Amino Acid	Protein*						
	Cyto	Hb alpha	Hb beta	RNase	Lys	Chgen	Fdox
Lysine	18	11	11	10	6	14	4
Histidine	3	10	9	4	1	2	1
Arginine	2	3	3	4	11	4	1
Aspartic acid**	8	12	13	15	21	23	13
Threonine	7	9	7	10	7	23	8
Serine	2	11	5	15	10	28	7

Amino Acid	Number of amino acids per protein molecule						
	Protein*						
	Cyto	Hb alpha	Hb beta	RNase	Lys	Chgen	Fdox
Glutamic acid**	10	5	11	12	5	15	13
Proline	4	7	7	4	2	9	4
Glycine	13	7	13	3	12	23	6
Alanine	6	21	15	12	12	22	9
Half-cystine	2	1	2	8	8	10	5
Valine	3	13	18	9	6	23	7
Methionine	3	2	1	4	2	2	0
Isoleucine	8	0	0	3	6	10	4
Leucine	6	18	18	2	8	19	8
Tyrosine	5	3	3	6	3	4	4
Phenylalanine	3	7	8	3	3	6	2
Tryptophan	1	1	2	0	6	8	1
Total	104	141	146	124	129	245	97

*Cyto = human cytochrome c; Hb alpha = human hemoglobin A, alpha-chain; Hb beta = human hemoglobin A, beta-chain; RNase = bovine ribonuclease; Lys = chicken lysozyme; Chgen = bovine chymotrypsinogen; Fdox = spinach ferredoxin.

**The values recorded for aspartic acid and glutamic acid include asparagine and glutamine, respectively.

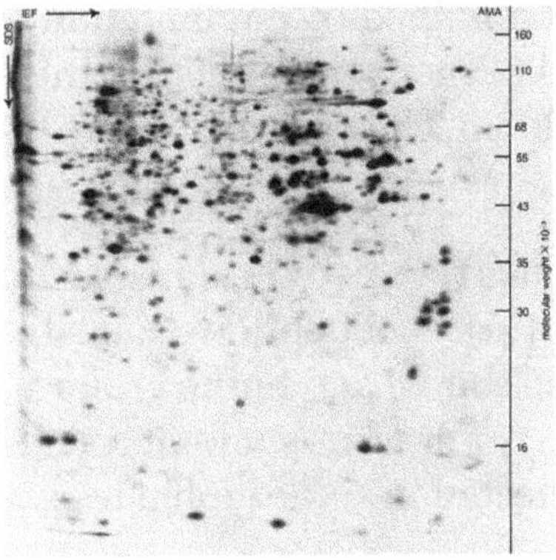

Two-dimensional gel electrophoresis

In figure, two-dimensional gel electrophoresis, proteins are separated based on charge and size. Approaches commonly employed include isoelectric focusing (IEF) sodium dodecyl sulfate (SDS) polyacrylamide gel electrophoresis (PAGE) and immobilized pH gradient (IPG-Dalt) SDS-PAGE.

Free-boundary electrophoresis, the original method of determining electrophoretic migration, has been replaced in many instances by zone electrophoresis, in which the protein is placed in either a gel of starch, agar, or polyacrylamide or in a porous medium such as paper or cellulose acetate. The migration of hemoglobin and other coloured proteins can be followed visually. Colourless proteins are made visible after the completion of electrophoresis by staining them with a suitable dye.

Conformation of Globular Proteins

Results of X-ray Diffraction Studies

Most knowledge concerning secondary and tertiary structure of globular proteins has been obtained by the examination of their crystals using X-ray diffraction. In this technique, X-rays are allowed to strike the crystal; the X-rays are diffracted by the crystal and impinge on a photographic plate, forming a pattern of spots. The measured intensity of the diffraction pattern, as recorded on a photographic film, depends particularly on the electron density of the atoms in the protein crystal. This density is lowest in hydrogen atoms, and they do not give a visible diffraction pattern. Although carbon, oxygen, and nitrogen atoms yield visible diffraction patterns, they are present in such great number-about 700 or 800 per 100 amino acids-that the resolution of the structure of a protein containing more than 100 amino acids is almost impossible. Resolution is considerably improved by substituting into the side chains of certain amino acids very heavy atoms, particularly those of heavy metals. Mercury ions, for example, bind to the sulfhydryl (-SH) groups of cysteine. Platinum chloride has been used in other proteins. In the iron-containing proteins, the iron atom already in the molecule is adequate.

Although the X-ray diffraction technique cannot resolve the complete three-dimensional conformation (that is, the secondary and tertiary structure of the peptide chain), complete resolution has been obtained by combination of the results of X-ray diffraction with those of amino acid sequence analysis. In this way the complete conformation of such proteins as myoglobin, chymotrypsinogen, lysozyme, and ribonuclease has been resolved.

The X-ray diffraction method has revealed regular structural arrangements in proteins; one is an extended form of antiparallel peptide chains that are linked to each other by hydrogen bonds between the carbonyl and imino groups. This conformation, called the pleated sheet, or β-structure, is found in some fibrous proteins. Short strands of the β-structure have also been detected in some globular proteins.

A second important structural arrangement is the α-helix; it is formed by a sequence of amino acids wound around a straight axis in either a right-handed or a left-handed spiral. Each turn of the helix corresponds to a distance of 5.4 angstroms (= 0.54 nanometre) in the direction of the screw axis and contains 3.7 amino acids. Hence, the length of the α-helix per amino acid residue is 5.4 divided by 3.7, or 1.5 angstroms

(1 angstrom = 0.1 nanometre). The stability of the α-helix is maintained by hydrogen bonds between the carbonyl and imino groups of neighbouring turns of the helix. It was once thought, based on data from analyses of the myoglobin molecule, more than half of which consists of α-helices, that the α-helix is the predominant structural element of the globular proteins; it is now known that myoglobin is exceptional in this respect. The other globular proteins for which the structures have been resolved by X-ray diffraction contain only small regions of α-helix. In most of them the peptide chains are folded in an apparently random fashion, for which the term random coil has been used. The term is misleading, however, because the folding is not random; rather, it is dictated by the primary structure and modified by the secondary and tertiary structures.

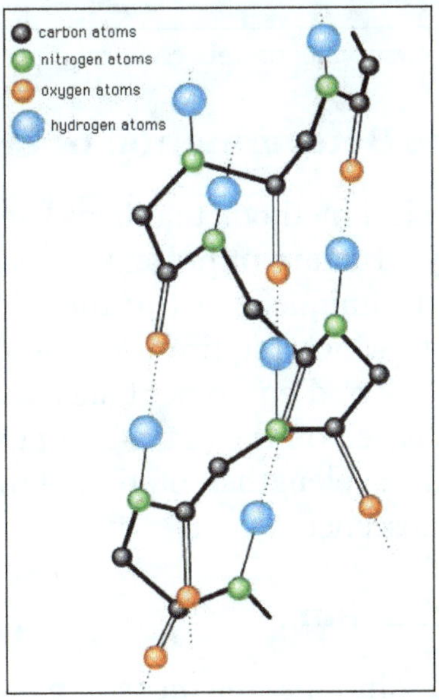

Protein structure (α-helix): The α-helix in the structural arrangement of a protein

The first proteins for which the internal structures were completely resolved are the iron-containing proteins myoglobin and hemoglobin. The investigation of the hydrated crystals of these proteins by Austrian-born British biochemist Max Perutz and British biochemist John C. Kendrew, revealed that the folding of the peptide chains is so tight that most of the water is displaced from the centre of the globular molecules. The amino acids that carry the ammonium ($-NH_3^+$) and carboxyl ($-COO^-$) groups were found to be shifted to the surface of the globular molecules, and the nonpolar amino acids were found to be concentrated in the interior.

The simplified structure of lysozyme from hen's egg white has a single peptide chain of 129 amino acids. The amino acid residues are numbered from the terminal α group (N) to the terminal carboxyl group (C). Circles indicate every fifth residue, and every tenth residue is numbered. Broken lines indicate the four disulfide bridges. Alpha-helices are visible in the ranges 25 to 35, 90 to 100, and 120 to 125.

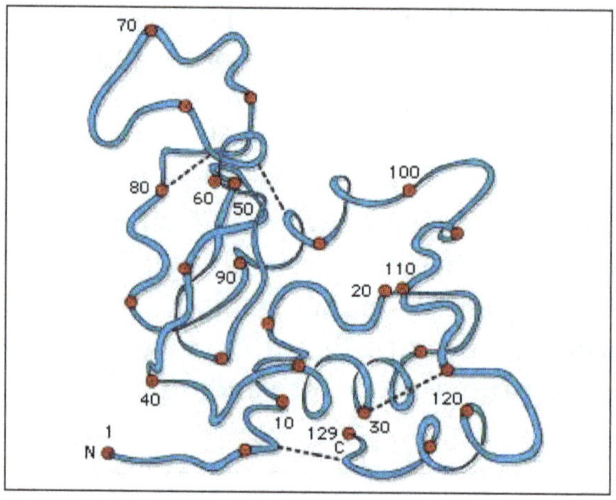

Lysozyme; protein conformation

Other Approaches to the Determination of Protein Structure

None of the several other physical methods that have been used to obtain information on the secondary and tertiary structure of proteins provides as much direct information as the X-ray diffraction technique. Most of the techniques, however, are much simpler than X-ray diffraction, which requires, for the resolution of the structure of one protein, many years of work and equipment such as electronic computers. Some of the simpler techniques are based on the optical properties of proteins—refractivity, absorption of light of different wavelengths, rotation of the plane polarized light at different wavelengths, and luminescence.

Spectrophotometric Behaviour

Spectrophotometry of protein solutions (the measurement of the degree of absorbance of light by a protein within a specified wavelength) is useful within the range of visible light only with proteins that contain coloured prosthetic groups (the nonprotein components). Examples of such proteins include the red heme proteins of the blood, the purple pigments of the retina of the eye, green and yellow proteins that contain bile pigments, blue copper-containing proteins, and dark brown proteins called melanins. Peptide bonds, because of their carbonyl groups, absorb light energy at very short wavelengths (185–200 nanometres). The aromatic rings of phenylalanine, tyrosine, and tryptophan, however, absorb ultraviolet light between wavelengths of 280 and 290 nanometres. The absorbance of ultraviolet light by tryptophan is greatest, that of tyrosine is less, and that of phenylalanine is least. If the tyrosine or tryptophan content of the protein is known, therefore, the concentration of the protein solution can be determined by measuring its absorbance between 280 and 290 nanometres.

Optical Activity

It will be recalled that the amino acids, with the exception of glycine, exhibit optical activity. It is not surprising, therefore, that proteins also are optically active. They are usually levorotatory (i.e., they rotate the plane of polarization to the left) when polarized light of wavelengths in the visible range is used. Although the specific rotation (a function of the concentration of a protein solution and the distance the light travels in it) of most L-amino acids varies from −30° to +30°, the amino acid cystine has a specific rotation of approximately −300°. Although the optical rotation of a protein depends on all of the amino acids of which it is composed, the most important ones are cystine and the aromatic amino acids phenylalanine, tyrosine, and tryptophan. The contribution of the other amino acids to the optical activity of a protein is negligibly small.

Chemical Reactivity of Proteins

Information on the internal structure of proteins can be obtained with chemical methods that reveal whether certain groups are present on the surface of the protein molecule and thus able to react or whether they are buried inside the closely folded peptide chains and thus are unable to react. The chemical reagents used in such investigations must be mild ones that do not affect the structure of the protein.

The reactivity of tyrosine is of special interest. It has been found, for example, that only three of the six tyrosines found in the naturally occurring enzyme ribonuclease can be iodinated (i.e., reacted to accept an iodine atom). Enzyme-catalyzed breakdown of iodinated ribonuclease is used to identify the peptides in which the iodinated tyrosines are present. The three tyrosines that can be iodinated lie on the surface of ribonuclease; the others, assumed to be inaccessible, are said to be buried in the molecule. Tyrosine can also be identified by using other techniques-e.g., treatment with diazonium compounds or tetranitromethane. Because the compounds formed are coloured, they can easily be detected when the protein is broken down with enzymes.

Cysteine can be detected by coupling with compounds such as iodoacetic acid or iodoacetamide; the reaction results in the formation of carboxymethylcysteine or carbamidomethylcysteine, which can be detected by amino acid determination of the peptides containing them. The imidazole groups of certain histidines can also be located by coupling with the same reagents under different conditions. Unfortunately, few other amino acids can be labelled without changes in the secondary and tertiary structure of the protein.

Association of Protein Subunits

Many proteins with molecular weights of more than 50,000 occur in aqueous solutions as complexes: dimers, tetramers, and higher polymers-i.e., as chains of two, four, or more repeating basic structural units. The subunits, which are called monomers or protomers, usually are present as an even number. Less than 10 percent of the polymers have been found to have an odd number of monomers. The arrangement of the subunits is thought to be regular and may be cyclic, cubic, or tetrahedral. Some of the small proteins also contain subunits. Insulin, for example, with a molecular weight of about 6,000, consists of two peptide chains linked to each other by disulfide bridges (-S-S-). Similar interchain disulfide bonds have been found in the immunoglobulins. In other proteins, hydrogen bonds and hydrophobic bonds (resulting from the interaction between the amino acid side chains of valine, leucine, isoleucine, and phenylalanine) cause the formation of aggregates of the subunits. The subunits of some proteins are identical; those of others differ. Hemoglobin is a tetramer consisting of two α-chains and two β-chains.

Protein Denaturation

When a solution of a protein is boiled, the protein frequently becomes insoluble—i.e., it is denatured—and remains insoluble even when the solution is cooled. The denaturation of the proteins of egg white by heat—as when boiling an egg—is an example of irreversible denaturation. The denatured protein has the same primary structure as the original, or native, protein. The weak forces between charged groups and the weaker forces of mutual attraction of nonpolar groups are disrupted at elevated temperatures, however; as a result, the tertiary structure of the protein is lost. In some instances the original structure of the protein can be regenerated; the process is called renaturation.

Denaturation can be brought about in various ways. Proteins are denatured by treatment with alkaline or acid, oxidizing or reducing agents, and certain organic solvents. Interesting among denaturing agents are those that affect the secondary and tertiary structure without affecting the primary structure. The agents most frequently used for this purpose are urea and guanidinium chloride. These molecules, because of their high affinity for peptide bonds, break the hydrogen bonds and the salt bridges between positive and negative side chains, thereby abolishing the tertiary structure of the peptide chain. When denaturing agents are removed from a protein solution, the native protein re-forms in many cases. Denaturation can also be accomplished by reduction of the disulfide bonds of cystine-i.e., conversion of the disulfide bond (-S-S-) to two sulfhydryl groups (-SH). This, results in the formation of two cysteines. Reoxidation of the cysteines by exposure to air sometimes regenerates the native protein. In other cases, however, the wrong cysteines become bound to each other, resulting in a different protein. Finally, denaturation can also be accomplished by exposing proteins to organic solvents such as ethanol or acetone. It is believed that the organic solvents interfere with the mutual attraction of nonpolar groups.

Some of the smaller proteins, however, are extremely stable, even against heat; for example, solutions of ribonuclease can be exposed for short periods of time to temperatures of 90 °C (194 °F) without undergoing significant denaturation. Denaturation does not involve identical changes in protein molecules. A common property of denatured proteins, however, is the loss of biological activity-e.g., the ability to act as enzymes or hormones.

Although denaturation had long been considered an all-or-none reaction, it is now thought that many intermediary states exist between native and denatured protein. In some instances, however, the breaking of a key bond could be followed by the complete breakdown of the conformation of the native protein.

Although many native proteins are resistant to the action of the enzyme trypsin, which breaks down proteins during digestion, they are hydrolyzed by the same enzyme after denaturation. The peptide bonds that can be split by trypsin are inaccessible in the native proteins but become accessible during denaturation. Similarly, denatured proteins give more intense colour reactions for tyrosine, histidine, and arginine than do the same proteins in the native state. The increased accessibility of reactive groups of denatured proteins is attributed to an unfolding of the peptide chains.

If denaturation can be brought about easily and if renaturation is difficult, how is the native conformation of globular proteins maintained in living organisms, in which they are produced stepwise, by incorporation of one amino acid at a time? Experiments on the biosynthesis of proteins from amino acids containing radioactive carbon or heavy hydrogen reveal that the protein molecule grows stepwise from the N terminus to the C terminus; in each step a single amino acid residue is incorporated. As soon as the growing peptide chain contains six or seven amino acid residues, the side chains interact with each other and thus cause deviations from the straight or β-chain configuration. Depending on the nature of the side chains, this may result in the formation of an α-helix or of loops closed by hydrogen bonds or disulfide bridges. The final conformation is probably frozen when the peptide chain attains a length of 50 or more amino acid residues.

Conformation of Proteins in Interfaces

Like many other substances with both hydrophilic and hydrophobic groups, soluble proteins tend to migrate into the interface between air and water or oil and water; the term oil here means a hydrophobic liquid such as benzene or xylene. Within the interface, proteins spread, forming thin films. Measurements of the surface tension, or interfacial tension, of such films indicate that tension is reduced by the protein film. Proteins, when forming an interfacial film, are present as a monomolecular layer-i.e., a layer one molecule in height. Although it was once thought that globular protein molecules unfold completely in the interface, it has now been established that many proteins can be recovered from films in the native state. The application of lateral pressure on a protein film causes it to increase in thickness and finally to form a layer with a height corresponding to the diameter of the native protein molecule. Protein molecules in an interface, because of Brownian motions (molecular vibrations), occupy much more space than do those in the film after the application of pressure. The Brownian motion of compressed molecules is limited to the two dimensions of the interface, since the protein molecules cannot move upward or downward.

The motion of protein molecules at the air–water interface has been used to determine the molecular weight of proteins. The technique involves measuring the force exerted by the protein layer on a barrier.

When a protein solution is vigorously shaken in air, it forms a foam, because the soluble proteins migrate into the air–water interface and persist there, preventing or slowing the reconversion of the foam into a homogeneous solution. Some of the unstable, easily modified proteins are denatured when spread in the air–water interface. The formation of a permanent foam when egg white is vigorously stirred is an example of irreversible denaturation by spreading in a surface.

Classification of Proteins

Classification by Solubility

After two German chemists, Emil Fischer and Franz Hofmeister, independently stated that proteins are essentially polypeptides consisting of many amino acids, an attempt was made to classify proteins according to their chemical and physical properties, because the biological function of proteins had not yet been established. Proteins were classified primarily according to their solubility in a number of solvents. This classification is no longer satisfactory, however, because proteins of quite different structure and function sometimes have similar solubilities; conversely, proteins of the same function and similar structure sometimes have different solubilities. The terms associated with the old classification, however, are still widely used.

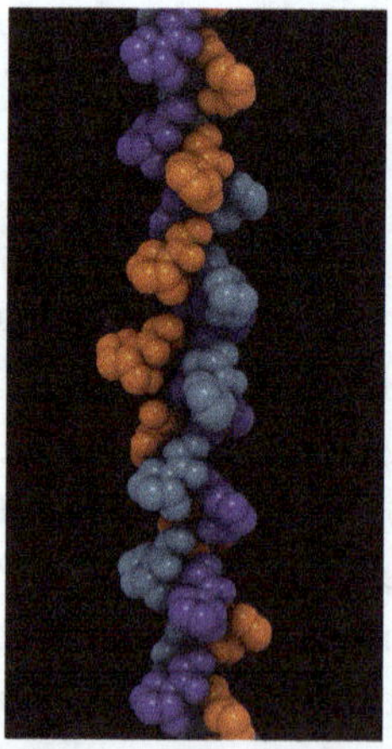

Collagen (Collagen molecule)

Albumins are proteins that are soluble in water and in water half-saturated with ammonium sulfate. On the other hand, globulins are salted out (i.e., precipitated) by half-saturation with ammonium sulfate. Globulins that are soluble in salt-free water are called pseudoglobulins; those insoluble in salt-free water are euglobulins. Both prolamins and glutelins, which are plant proteins, are insoluble in water; the prolamins dissolve in 50 to 80 percent ethanol, the glutelins in acidified or alkaline solution. The term protamine is used for a number of proteins in fish sperm that consist of approximately 80 percent arginine and therefore are strongly alkaline. Histones, which are less alkaline, apparently occur only in cell nuclei, where they are bound to nucleic acids. The term scleroproteins has been used for the insoluble proteins of animal organs. They include keratin, the insoluble protein of certain epithelial tissues such as the skin or hair, and collagen, the protein of the connective tissue. A large group of proteins has been called conjugated proteins, because they are complex molecules of protein consisting of protein and nonprotein moieties. The nonprotein portion is called the prosthetic group. Conjugated proteins can be subdivided into mucoproteins, which, in addition to protein, contain carbohydrate; lipoproteins, which contain lipids; phosphoproteins, which are rich in phosphate; chromoproteins, which contain pigments such as iron-porphyrins, carotenoids, bile pigments, and melanin; and finally, nucleoproteins, which contain nucleic acid.

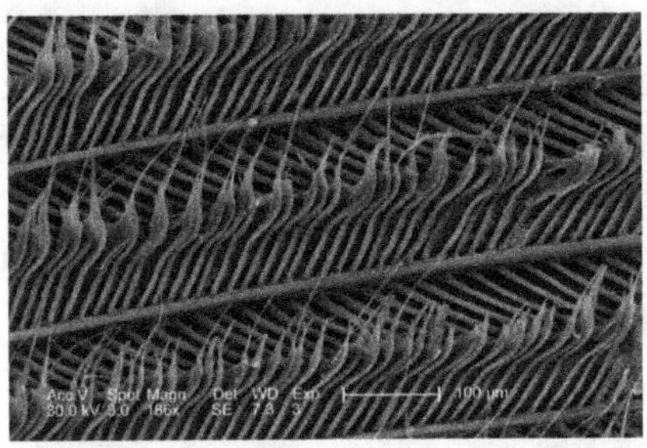

Keratin: Scanning electron micrograph showing strands of keratin in a feather

The weakness of the above classification lies in the fact that many, if not all, globulins contain small amounts of carbohydrate; thus there is no sharp borderline between globulins and mucoproteins. Moreover, the phosphoproteins do not have a prosthetic group that can be isolated; they are merely proteins in which some of the hydroxyl groups of serine are phosphorylated (i.e., contain phosphate). Finally, the globulins include proteins with quite different roles-enzymes, antibodies, fibrous proteins, and contractile proteins.

Classification by Biological Functions

In view of the unsatisfactory state of the old classification, it is preferable to classify the proteins according to their biological function. Such a classification is far from ideal, however, because one protein can have more than one function. The contractile protein myosin, for example, also acts as an ATPase (adenosine triphosphatase), an enzyme that hydrolyzes adenosine triphosphate (removes a phosphate group from ATP by introducing a water molecule). Another problem with functional classification is that the definite function of a protein frequently is not known. A protein cannot be called an enzyme as long as its substrate (the specific compound upon which it acts) is not known. It cannot even be tested for its enzymatic action when its substrate is not known.

Special Structure and Function of Proteins

Despite its weaknesses, a functional classification is used here in order to demonstrate, whenever possible, the correlation between the structure and function of a protein. The structural, fibrous proteins are presented first, because their structure is simpler than that of the globular proteins and more clearly related to their function, which is the maintenance of either a rigid or a flexible structure.

Structural Proteins: Scleroproteins

Collagen

Collagen is the structural protein of bones, tendons, ligaments, and skin. For many years collagen was considered to be insoluble in water. Part of the collagen of calf skin, however, can be extracted with citrate buffer at pH 3.7. A precursor of collagen called procollagen is converted in the body into collagen. Procollagen has a molecular weight of 120,000. Cleavage of one or a few peptide bonds of procollagen yields collagen, which has three subunits, each with a molecular weight of 95,000; therefore, the molecular weight of collagen is 285,000 (3 × 95,000). The three subunits are wound as spirals around an elongated straight axis. The length of each subunit is 2,900 angstroms, and its diameter is approximately 15 angstroms. The three chains are staggered, so that the trimer has no definite terminal limits.

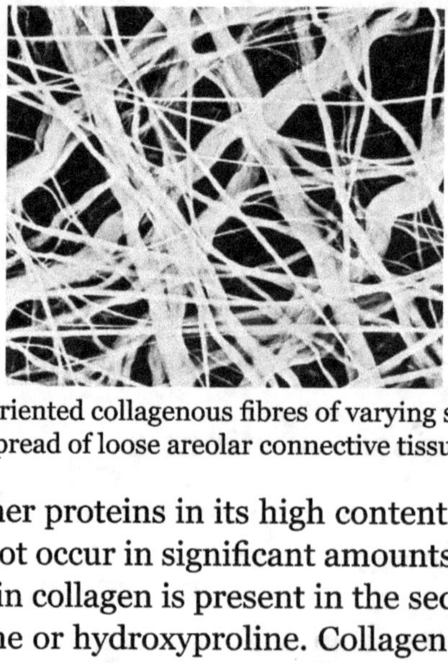

Randomly oriented collagenous fibres of varying size in a thin spread of loose areolar connective tissue

Collagen differs from all other proteins in its high content of proline and hydroxyproline. Hydroxyproline does not occur in significant amounts in any other protein except elastin. Most of the proline in collagen is present in the sequence glycine-proline-X, in which X is frequently alanine or hydroxyproline. Collagen does not contain cystine or tryptophan and therefore cannot substitute for other proteins in the diet. The presence of proline causes kinks in the peptide chain and thus reduces the length of the amino acid unit from 3.7 angstroms in the extended chain of the β-structure to 2.86 angstroms in the collagen chain. In the intertwined triple helix, the glycines are inside, close to the axis; the prolines are outside.

Native collagen resists the action of trypsin but is hydrolyzed by the bacterial enzyme collagenase. When collagen is boiled with water, the triple helix is destroyed, and the subunits are partially hydrolyzed; the product is gelatin. The unfolded peptide chains of gelatin trap large amounts of water, resulting in a hydrated molecule.

When collagen is treated with tannic acid or with chromium salts, cross links form between the collagen fibres, and it becomes insoluble; the conversion of hide into leather is based on this tanning process. The tanned material is insoluble in hot water and cannot be converted to gelatin. On exposure to water at 62° to 63 °C (144° to 145 °F), however, the cross links formed by the tanning agents collapse, and the leather contracts irreversibly to about one-third its original volume.

Collagen seems to undergo an aging process in living organisms that may be caused by the formation of cross links between collagen fibres. They are formed by the conversion of some lysine side chains to aldehydes (compounds with the general structure RCHO), and the combination of the aldehydes with the ε-amino groups of intact lysine side chains. The protein elastin, which occurs in the elastic fibres of connective tissue, contains similar cross links and may result from the combination of collagen fibres with other proteins. When cross-linked collagen or elastin is degraded, products of the cross-linked lysine fragments, called desmosins and isodesmosins, are formed.

Keratin

Keratin, the structural protein of epithelial cells in the outermost layers of the skin, has been isolated from hair, nails, hoofs, and feathers. Keratin is completely insoluble in cold or hot water; it is not attacked by proteolytic enzymes (i.e., enzymes that break apart, or lyse, protein molecules), and therefore cannot replace proteins in the diet. The great stability of keratin results from the numerous disulfide bonds of cystine. The amino acid composition of keratin differs from that of collagen. Cystine may account for 24 percent of the total amino acids. The peptide chains of keratin are arranged in approximately equal amounts of antiparallel and parallel pleated sheets, in which the peptide chains are linked to each other by hydrogen bonds between the carbonyl and imino groups.

Reduction of the disulfide bonds to sulfhydryl groups results in dissociation of the peptide chains, the molecular weight of which is 25,000 to 28,000 each. The formation of permanent waves in the beauty treatment of hair is based on partial reduction of the disulfide bonds of hair keratin by thioglycol, or some other mild reducing agent, and subsequent oxidation of the sulfhydryl groups (-SH) in the reoriented hair to disulfide bonds (-S-S-) by exposure to the oxygen of the air.

The length of keratin fibres depends on their water content. They can bind approximately 16 percent of water; this hydration is accompanied by an increase in the length of the fibres of 10 to 12 percent.

The most thoroughly investigated keratin is hair keratin, particularly that of wool. It consists of a mixture of peptides with high and low cystine content. When wool is heated in water to about 90° C (190° F), it shrinks irreversibly. This is attributed to the breakage of hydrogen bonds and other noncovalent bonds; disulfide bonds do not seem to be affected.

Others

The most thoroughly investigated scleroprotein has been fibroin, the insoluble material of silk. The raw silk comprising the cocoon of the silkworm consists of two proteins. One, sericin, is soluble in hot water; the other, fibroin, is not. The amino acid composition of the latter differs from that of all other proteins. It contains large amounts of glycine, alanine, tyrosine, and serine; small amounts of the other amino acids; and no sulfur-containing ones. The peptide chains are arranged in antiparallel β-structures. Fibroin is partly soluble in concentrated solutions of lithium thiocyanate or in mixtures of cupric salts and ethylene diamine. Such solutions contain a protein of molecular weight 170,000, which is a dimer of two subunits.

Little is known about either the scleroproteins of the marine sponges or the insoluble proteins of the cellular membranes of animal cells. Some of the membranes are soluble in detergents; others, however, are detergent-insoluble.

The Muscle Proteins

The total amount of muscle proteins in mammals, including humans, exceeds that of any other protein. About 40 percent of the body weight of a healthy human adult weighing about 70 kilograms (150 pounds) is muscle, which is composed of about 20 percent muscle protein. Thus, the human body contains about 5 to 6 kilograms (11 to 13 pounds) of muscle protein. An albumin-like fraction of these proteins, originally called myogen, contains various enzymes—phosphorylase, aldolase, glyceraldehyde phosphate dehydrogenase, and others; it does not seem to be involved in contraction. The globulin fraction contains myosin, the contractile protein, which also occurs in blood platelets, small bodies found in blood. Similar contractile substances occur in other contractile structures; for example, in the cilia or flagella (whiplike organs of locomotion) of bacteria and protozoans. In contrast to the scleroproteins, the contractile proteins are soluble in salt solutions and susceptible to enzymatic digestion.

The energy required for muscle contraction is provided by the oxidation of carbohydrates or lipids. The term mechanochemical reaction has been used for this conversion of chemical into mechanical energy. The molecular process underlying the reaction is known to involve the fibrous muscle proteins, the peptide chains of which undergo a change in conformation during contraction.

Myosin, which can be removed from fresh muscle by adding it to a chilled solution of dilute potassium chloride and sodium bicarbonate, is insoluble in water. Myosin, solutions of which are highly viscous, consists of an elongated-probably double-stranded-peptide chain, which is coiled at both ends in such a way that a terminal globule is formed. The length of the molecule is approximately 160 nanometres and its average diameter 2.6 nanometres. The equivalent weight of each of the two terminal globules is approximately 30,000; the molecular weight of myosin is close to 500,000. Trypsin splits myosin into large fragments called meromyosin. Myosin contains many amino acids with positively and negatively charged side chains; they form 18 and 16 percent, respectively, of the total number of amino acids. Myosin catalyzes the hydrolytic cleavage of ATP (adenosine triphosphate). A smaller protein with properties similar to those of myosin is tropomyosin. It has a molecular weight of 70,000 and dimensions of 45 by 2 nanometres. More than 90 percent of its peptide chains are present in the α-helix form.

Myosin combines easily with another muscle protein called actin, the molecular weight of which is about 50,000; it forms 12 to 15 percent of the muscle proteins. Actin can exist in two forms-one, G-actin, is globular; the other, F-actin, is fibrous. Actomyosin is a complex molecule formed by one molecule of myosin and one or two molecules of actin. In muscle, actin and myosin filaments are oriented parallel to each other and to the long axis of the muscle. The actin filaments are linked to each other lengthwise by fine threads called S filaments. During contraction the S filaments shorten, so that the actin filaments slide toward each other, past the myosin filaments, thus causing a shortening of the muscle.

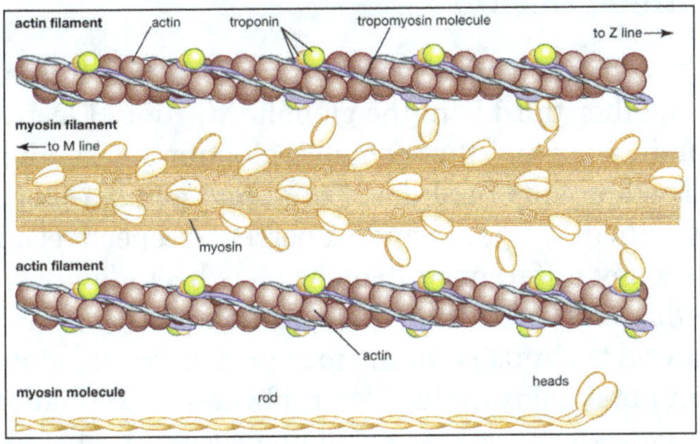

Muscle (actin and myosin): The structure of actin and myosin filaments

Fibrinogen and Fibrin

Fibrinogen, the protein of the blood plasma, is converted into the insoluble protein fibrin during the clotting process. The fibrinogen-free fluid obtained after removal of the clot, called blood serum, is blood plasma minus fibrinogen. The fibrinogen content of the blood plasma is 0.2 to 0.4 percent.

Fibrinogen can be precipitated from the blood plasma by half-saturation with sodium chloride. Fibrinogen solutions are highly viscous and show strong flow birefringence. In electron micrographs the molecules appear as rods with a length of 47.5 nanometres and a diameter of 1.5 nanometres; in addition, two terminal and a central nodule are visible. The molecular weight is 340,000. An unusually high percentage, about 36 percent, of the amino acid side chains are positively or negatively charged.

The clotting process is initiated by the enzyme thrombin, which catalyzes the breakage of a few peptide bonds of fibrinogen; as a result, two small fibrinopeptides with molecular weights of 1,900 and 2,400 are released. The remainder of the fibrinogen molecule, a monomer, is soluble and stable at pH values less than 6 (i.e., in acid solutions). In neutral solution (pH 7) the monomer is converted into a larger molecule, insoluble fibrin; this results from the formation of new peptide bonds. The newly formed peptide bonds form intermolecular and intramolecular cross links, thus giving rise to a large clot, in which all molecules are linked to each other. Clotting, which takes place only in the presence of calcium ions, can be prevented by compounds such as oxalate or citrate, which have a high affinity for calcium ions.

Albumins, Globulins and other Soluble Proteins

The blood plasma, the lymph, and other animal fluids usually contain one to seven grams of protein per 100 millilitres of fluid, which includes small amounts of hundreds of enzymes and a large number of protein hormones.

Proteins of the Blood Serum

Human blood serum contains about 7 percent protein, two-thirds of which is in the albumin fraction; the other third is in the globulin fraction. Electrophoresis of serum reveals a large albumin peak and three smaller globulin peaks, the alpha-, beta-, and gamma-globulins. The amounts of alpha-, beta-, and gamma-globulin in normal human serum are approximately 1.5, 1.9, and 1.1 percent, respectively. Each globulin fraction is a mixture of many different proteins, as has been demonstrated by immunoelectrophoresis. In this method, serum from an animal (e.g., a rabbit) injected with human serum is allowed to diffuse into the four protein bands-albumin, alpha-, beta-, and gamma-globulin-obtained from the electrophoresis of human serum. Because the animal has previously been injected with human serum, its blood contains antibodies (substances formed in response to a foreign substance introduced into the body) against each of the human serum proteins; each antibody combines with the serum protein (antigen) that caused its formation in the animal. The result is the formation of about 20 regions of insoluble antigen-antibody precipitate, which appear as white arcs in the transparent gel of the electrophoresis medium. Each region corresponds to a different human serum protein.

Serum albumin is much less heterogeneous (i.e., contains fewer distinct proteins) than are the globulins; in fact, it is one of the few serum proteins that can be obtained in a crystalline form. Serum albumin combines easily with many acidic dyes (e.g., Congo red and methyl orange); with bilirubin, the yellow bile pigment; and with fatty acids. It seems to act, in living organisms, as a carrier for certain biological substances. Present in blood serum in relatively high concentration, serum albumin also acts as a protective colloid, a protein that stabilizes other proteins. Albumin (molecular weight of 68,000) has a single free sulfhydryl (- SH) group, which on oxidation forms a disulfide bond with the sulfhydryl group of another serum albumin molecule, thus forming a dimer. The isoelectric point of serum albumin is pH 4.7.

The alpha-globulin fraction of blood serum is a mixture of several conjugated proteins. The best known are an α-lipoprotein (combination of lipid and protein) and two mucoproteins (combinations of carbohydrate and protein). One mucoprotein is called orosomucoid, or α1-acid glycoprotein; the other is called haptoglobin because it combines specifically with globin, the protein component of hemoglobin. Haptoglobin contains about 20 percent carbohydrate. The beta-globulin fraction of serum contains, in addition to lipoproteins and mucoproteins, two metal-binding proteins, transferrin and ceruloplasmin, which bind iron and copper, respectively. They are the principal iron and copper carriers of the blood.

The gamma-globulins are the most heterogeneous globulins. Although most have a molecular weight of approximately 150,000, that of some, called macroglobulins, is as high as 800,000. Because typical antibodies are of the same size and exhibit the same electrophoretic behaviour as γ-globulins, they are called immunoglobulins. The designation IgM or gamma M (γM) is used for the macroglobulins; the designation IgG or gamma G (γG) is used for γ–globulins of molecular weight 150,000.

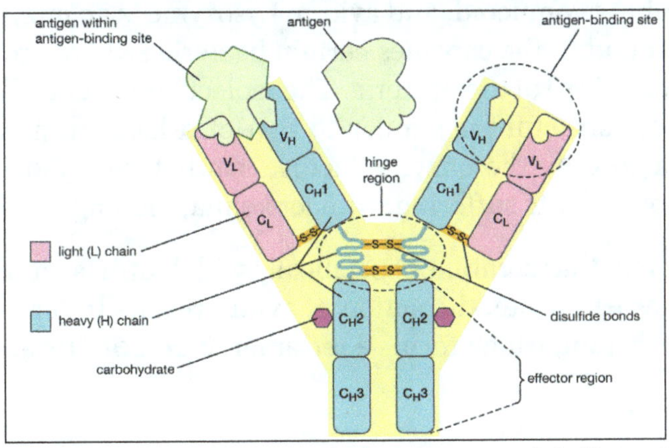

The four-chain structure of an antibody, or immunoglobulin, molecule

In figure, the basic unit is composed of two identical light (L) chains and two identical heavy (H) chains, which are held together by disulfide bonds to form a flexible Y shape. Each chain is composed of a variable (V) region and a constant (C) region.

Milk Proteins

Milk contains the following: an albumin, α-lactalbumin; a globulin, beta-lactoglobulin; and a phosphoprotein, casein. If acid is added to milk, casein precipitates. The remaining watery liquid (the supernatant solution), or whey, contains α-lactalbumin and β-lactoglobulin. Both have been obtained in crystalline form; in bovine milk, their molecular weights are approximately 14,000 and 18,400, respectively. Lactoglobulin also occurs as a dimer of molecular weight 37,000. Genetic variations can produce small variations in the amino acid composition of lactoglobulin. The amino acid composition and the tertiary structure of lactalbumin resemble that of lysozyme, an egg protein.

Casein is precipitated not only by the addition of acid but also by the action of the enzyme rennin, which is found in gastric juice. Rennin from calf stomachs is used to precipitate casein, from which cheese is made. Milk fat precipitates with casein; milk sugar, however, remains in the supernatant (whey). Casein is a mixture of several similar phosphoproteins, called α-, β-, γ–, and κ-casein, all of which contain some serine side chains combined with phosphoric acid. Approximately 75 percent of casein is α-casein. Cystine has been found only in κ-casein. In milk, casein seems to form polymeric globules (micelles) with radially arranged monomers, each with a molecular weight of 24,000; the acidic side chains occur predominantly on the surface of the micelle, rather than inside.

Egg Proteins

About 50 percent of the proteins of egg white are composed of ovalbumin, which is easily obtained in crystals. Its molecular weight is 46,000 and its amino acid composition differs from that of serum albumin. Other proteins of egg white are conalbumin, lysozyme, ovoglobulin, ovomucoid, and avidin. Lysozyme is an enzyme that hydrolyzes the carbohydrates found in the capsules certain bacteria secrete around themselves; it causes lysis (disintegration) of the bacteria. The molecular weight of lysozyme is 14,100. Its three-dimensional structure is similar to that of α-lactalbumin, which stimulates the formation of lactose by the enzyme lactose synthetase. Lysozyme has also been found in the urine of patients suffering from leukemia, meningitis, and renal disease.

Avidin is a glycoprotein that combines specifically with biotin, a vitamin. In animals fed large amounts of raw egg white, the action of avidin results in "egg-white injury." The molecular weight of avidin, which forms a tetramer, is 16,200. Its amino acid sequence is known.

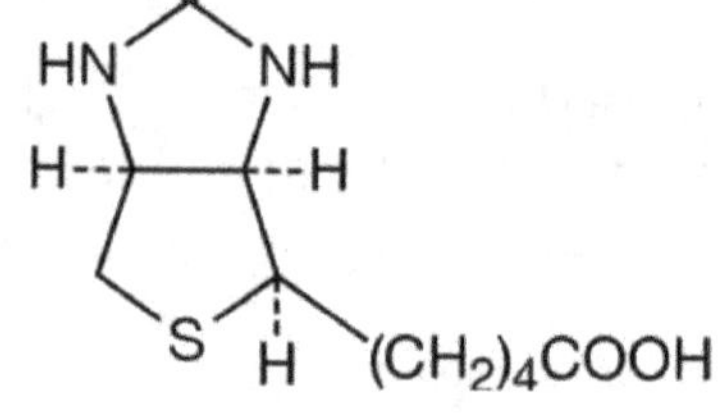

Egg-yolk proteins contain a mixture of lipoproteins and livetins. The latter are similar to serum albumin, α-globulin, and β-globulin. The yolk also contains a phosphoprotein, phosvitin. Phosvitin, which has also been found in fish sperm, has a molecular weight of 40,000 and an unusual amino acid composition; one third of its amino acids are phosphoserine.

Protamines and Histones

Protamines are found in the sperm cells of fish. The most thoroughly investigated protamines are salmine from salmon sperm and clupeine from herring sperm. The protamines are bound to deoxyribonucleic acid (DNA), forming nucleoprotamines. The amino acid composition of the protamines is simple; they contain, in addition to large amounts of arginine, small amounts of five or six other amino acids. The composition of the salmine molecule, for example, is: Arg_{51}, Ala_4, Val_4, Ile_1, Pro_7, and Ser_6, in which the subscript numbers indicate the number of each amino acid in the molecule. Because of the high arginine content, the isoelectric points of the protamines are at pH values of 11 to 12; i.e., the protamines are alkaline. The molecular weights of salmine and clupeine are close to 6,000. All of the protamines investigated thus far are mixtures of several similar proteins.

The histones are less basic than the protamines. They contain high amounts of either lysine or arginine and small amounts of aspartic acid and glutamic acid. Histones occur in combination with DNA as nucleohistones in the nuclei of the body cells of animals and plants, but not in animal sperm. The molecular weights of histones vary from 10,000 to 22,000. In contrast to the protamines, the histones contain most of the 20 amino acids, with the exception of tryptophan and the sulfur-containing ones. Like the protamines, histone preparations are heterogeneous mixtures. The amino acid sequence of some of the histones has been determined.

Plant Proteins

Plant proteins, mostly globulins, have been obtained chiefly from the protein-rich seeds of cereals and legumes. Small amounts of albumins are found in seeds. The best known globulins, insoluble in water, can be extracted from seeds by treatment with 2 to 10 percent solutions of sodium chloride. Many plant globulins have been obtained in crystalline form; they include edestin from hemp, molecular weight 310,000; amandin from almonds, 330,000; concanavalin A (42,000) and B (96,000); and canavalin (113,000) from jack beans. They are polymers of smaller subunits; edestin, for example, is a hexamer of a subunit with a molecular weight of 50,000, and concanavalin B a trimer of a subunit with a molecular weight of 30,000. After extraction of lipids from cereal seeds by ether and alcohol, further extraction with water containing 50 to 80 percent of alcohol yields proteins that are insoluble in water but soluble in water–ethanol mixtures and have been called prolamins. Their solubility in aqueous ethanol may result from their high proline and glutamine content. Gliadin, the prolamin from wheat, contains 14 grams of proline and 46 grams of glutamic acid in 100 grams of protein; most of the glutamic acid is in the form of glutamine. The total amounts of the basic amino acids (arginine, lysine, and histidine) in gliadin are only 5 percent of the weight of gliadin. Because the glysine content is either low or nonexistent, human populations dependent on grain as a sole protein source suffer from lysine deficiency.

Conjugated Proteins

Combination of Proteins with Prosthetic Groups

The link between a protein molecule and its prosthetic group is a covalent bond (an electron-sharing bond) in the glycoproteins, the biliproteins, and some of the heme proteins. In lipoproteins, nucleoproteins, and some heme proteins, the two components are linked by noncovalent bonds; the bonding results from the same forces that are responsible for the tertiary structure of proteins: hydrogen bonds, salt bridges between positively and negatively charged groups, disulfide bonds, and mutual interaction of hydrophobic groups. In the metalloproteins (proteins with a metal element as a prosthetic group), the metal ion usually forms a centre to which various groups are bound.

Some of the conjugated proteins have been mentioned in preceding sections because they occur in the blood serum, in milk, and in eggs.

Mucoproteins and Glycoproteins

The prosthetic groups in mucoproteins and glycoproteins are oligosaccharides (carbohydrates consisting of a small number of simple sugar molecules) usually containing from four to 12 sugar molecules; the most common sugars are galactose, mannose, glucosamine, and galactosamine. Xylose, fucose, glucuronic acid, sialic acid, and other simple sugars sometimes also occur. Some mucoproteins contain 20 percent or more of carbohydrate, usually in several oligosaccharides attached to different parts of the peptide chain. The designation mucoprotein is used for proteins with more than 3 to 4 percent carbohydrate; if the carbohydrate content is less than 3 percent, the protein is sometimes called a glycoprotein or simply a protein.

Mucoproteins, highly viscous proteins originally called mucins, are found in saliva, in gastric juice, and in other animal secretions. Mucoproteins occur in large amounts in cartilage, synovial fluid (the lubricating fluid of joints and tendons), and egg white. The mucoprotein of cartilage is formed by the combination of collagen with chondroitinsulfuric acid, which is a polymer of either glucuronic or iduronic acid and acetylhexosamine or acetylgalactosamine. It is not yet clear whether or not chondroitinsulfate is bound to collagen by covalent bonds.

Lipoproteins and Proteolipids

The bond between the protein and the lipid portion of lipoproteins and proteolipids is a noncovalent one. It is thought that some of the lipid is enclosed in a meshlike arrangement of peptide chains and becomes accessible for reaction only after the unfolding of the chains by denaturing agents. Although lipoproteins in the α- and β-globulin fraction of blood serum are soluble in water (but insoluble in organic solvents), some of the brain lipoproteins, because they have a high lipid content, are soluble in organic solvents; they are called proteolipids. The β-lipoprotein of human blood serum is a macroglobulin with a molecular weight of about 1,300,000, 70 percent of which is lipid; of the lipid, about 30 percent is phospholipid and 40 percent cholesterol and compounds derived from it. Because of their lipid content, the lipoproteins have the lowest density (mass per unit volume) of all proteins and are usually classified as low- and high-density lipoproteins (LDL and HDL).

Coloured lipoproteins are formed by the combination of protein with carotenoids. Crustacyanin, the pigment of lobsters, crayfish, and other crustaceans, contains astaxanthin, which is a compound derived from carotene. Among the most interesting of the coloured lipoproteins are the pigments of the retina of the eye. They contain retinal, which is a compound derived from carotene and which is formed by the oxidation of vitamin A. In rhodopsin, the red pigment of the retina, the aldehyde group (-CHO) of retinal forms a covalent bond with an amino ($-NH_2$) group of opsin, the protein carrier. Colour vision is mediated by the presence of several visual pigments in the retina that differ from rhodopsin either in the structure of retinal or in that of the protein carrier.

Metalloproteins

Proteins in which heavy metal ions are bound directly to some of the side chains of histidine, cysteine, or some other amino acid are called metalloproteins. Two metalloproteins, transferrin and ceruloplasmin, occur in the globulin fractions of blood serum; they act as carriers of iron and copper, respectively. Transferrin has a molecular weight of about 80,000 and consists of two identical subunits, each of which contains one ferric ion (Fe^{3+}) that seems to be bound to tyrosine. Several genetic variants of transferrin are known to occur in humans. Another iron protein, ferritin, which contains 20 to 22 percent iron, is the form in which iron is stored in animals; it has been obtained in crystalline form from liver and spleen. A molecule consisting of 20 subunits, its molecular weight is approximately 480,000. The iron can be removed by reduction from the ferric (Fe^{3+}) to the ferrous (Fe^{2+}) state. The iron-free protein, apoferritin, is synthesized in the body before the iron is incorporated.

Green plants and some photosynthetic and nitrogen-fixing bacteria (i.e., bacteria that convert atmospheric nitrogen, N_2, into amino acids and proteins) contain various ferredoxins. They are small proteins containing 50 to 100 amino acids and a chain of iron and disulfide units (FeS_2), in which some of the sulfur atoms are contributed by cysteine; others are sulfide ions (S^{2-}). The number of FeS_2 units per ferredoxin molecule varies from five in the ferredoxin of spinach to 10 in the ferredoxin of certain bacteria. Ferredoxins act as electron carriers in photosynthesis and in nitrogen fixation.

Ceruloplasmin is a copper-containing globulin that has a molecular weight of 151,000; the molecule consists of eight subunits, each containing one copper ion. Ceruloplasmin is the principal carrier of copper in organisms, although copper can also be transported by the iron-containing globulin transferrin. Another copper-containing protein, copper-zinc superoxide dismutase (formerly known as erythrocuprein), has been isolated from red blood cells; it has also been found in the liver and in the brain. The molecule, which consists of two subunits of similar size, contains copper ions and zinc ions. Because of their copper content, ceruloplasmin and copper-zinc superoxide dismutase possess catalytic activity in oxidation-reduction reactions.

Many animal enzymes contain zinc ions, which are usually bound to the sulfur of cysteine.

Horse kidneys contain the protein metallothionein, which contain zinc and cadmium; both are bound to sulfur. A vanadium-protein complex (hemovanadin) has been found in surprisingly high amounts in yellowish-green cells (vanadocytes) of tunicates, which are marine invertebrates.

Heme Proteins and other Chromoproteins

Although the heme proteins contain iron, they are usually not classified as metalloproteins, because their prosthetic group is an iron-porphyrin complex in which the iron is bound very firmly. The intense red or brown colour of the heme proteins is not caused by iron but by porphyrin, a complex cyclic structure. All porphyrin compounds absorb light intensely at or close to 410 nanometres. Porphyrin consists of four pyrrole rings (five-membered closed structures containing one nitrogen and four carbon atoms) linked to each other by methine groups (-CH=). The iron atom is kept in the centre of the porphyrin ring by interaction with the four nitrogen atoms. The iron atom can combine with two other substituents; in oxyhemoglobin, one substituent is a histidine of the protein carrier, the other is an oxygen molecule. In some heme proteins, the protein is also bound covalently to the side chains of porphyrin.

The chromoprotein melanin, a pigment found in dark skin, dark hair, and melanotic tumours, occurs in every major group of living organisms and appears to be remarkably diverse in structure. In humans, melanin produced by melanocytes may be dark brown (eumelanin) or pale red or yellowish (phaeomelanin). The different types are synthesized via different pathways, though they share the same initial step—the oxidation of tyrosine.

Green chromoproteins called biliproteins are found in many insects, such as grasshoppers, and also in the eggshells of many birds. The biliproteins are derived from the bile pigment biliverdin, which in turn is formed from porphyrin; biliverdin contains four pyrrole rings and three of the four methine groups of porphyrin. Large amounts of biliproteins have been found in red algae and blue-green algae; the red protein is called phycoerythrin, the blue one phycocyanobilin.

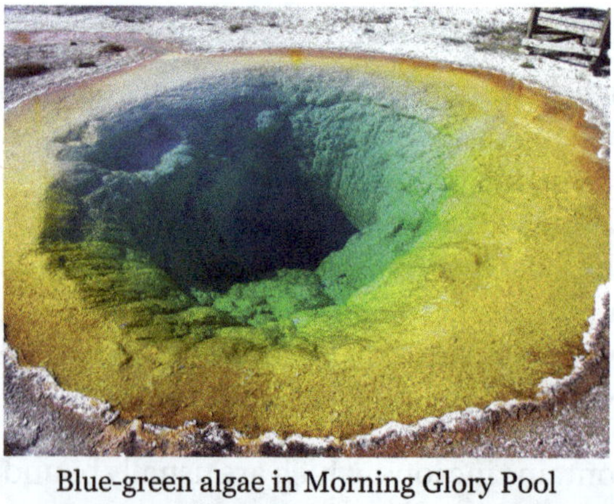

Blue-green algae in Morning Glory Pool

Nucleoproteins

When a protein solution is mixed with a solution of a nucleic acid, the phosphoric acid component of the nucleic acid combines with the positively charged ammonium groups ($-NH_3^+$) of the protein to form a protein–nucleic acid complex. The nucleus of a cell contains predominantly deoxyribonucleic acid (DNA) and the cytoplasm predominantly ribonucleic acid (RNA); both parts of the cell also contain protein. Protein–nucleic acid complexes, therefore, form in living cells.

The only nucleoproteins for which some evidence for specificity exists are nucleoprotamines, nucleohistones, and some RNA and DNA viruses. The nucleoprotamines are the form in which protamines occur in the sperm cells of fish; the histones of the thymus and of pea seedlings and other plant material apparently occur predominantly as nucleohistones. Both nucleoprotamines and nucleohistones contain only DNA.

Some of the simplest viruses consist of a specific RNA, which is coated by protein. One of the best known RNA viruses, tobacco mosaic virus (TMV), has the shape of a rod. RNA comprises only 5.1 percent of the mass of the virus. The complete sequence of the virus protein, which consists of about 2,130 identical peptide chains, each containing 158 amino acids, has been determined. The protein is arranged in a spiral around the RNA core.

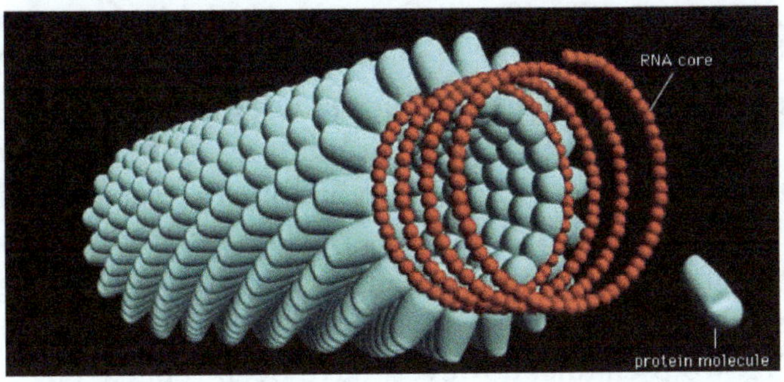

Schematic structure of the tobacco mosaic virus: The cutaway section shows the helical ribonucleic acid associated with protein molecules in a ratio of three nucleotides per protein molecule

DNA has been found in most bacterial viruses (bacteriophages) and in some animal viruses. As in TMV, the core of DNA is surrounded by protein. Phage protein is a mixture of enzymes and therefore cannot be considered as the protein portion of only one nucleoprotein.

Respiratory Proteins

Hemoglobin

Hemoglobin is the oxygen carrier in all vertebrates and some invertebrates. In oxyhemoglobin (HbO_2), which is bright red, the ferrous ion (Fe^{2+}) is bound to the four nitrogen atoms of porphyrin; the other two substituents are an oxygen molecule and the histidine of globin, the protein component of hemoglobin. Deoxyhemoglobin (deoxy-Hb), as its name implies, is oxyhemoglobin minus oxygen (i.e., reduced hemoglobin); it is purple in colour. Oxidation of the ferrous ion of hemoglobin yields a ferric compound, methemoglobin, sometimes called hemiglobin or ferrihemoglobin. The oxygen of oxyhemoglobin can be displaced by carbon monoxide, for which hemoglobin has a much greater affinity, preventing oxygen from reaching the body tissues.

The hemoglobins of all mammals, birds, and many other vertebrates are tetramers of two α- and two β-chains. The molecular weight of the tetramer is 64,500; the molecular weight of the α- and β-chains is approximately 16,100 each, and the four subunits are linked to each other by noncovalent interactions. If hemin (the ferric porphyrin component) is removed from globin (the protein component), two molecules of globin, each consisting of one α- and one β-chain, are obtained; the molecular weight of globin is 32,200. In contrast to hemoglobin, globin is an unstable protein that is easily denatured. If native globin is incubated with a solution of hemin at pH values of 8 to 9, native hemoglobin is reconstituted. Myoglobin, the red pigment of mammalian muscles, is a monomer with a molecular weight of 16,000.

The mammalian hemoglobins differ from each other in their amino acid composition and therefore in their secondary and tertiary structure. Rat and horse hemoglobins crystallize very easily, but those of humans, cattle, and sheep, because they are more soluble, are difficult to crystallize. The shape of hemoglobin crystals varies in different species; moreover, decomposition and denaturation occur at different rates in different species. It was also found that the blood of human newborns contains two different hemoglobins: about 20 percent of their hemoglobin is an adult hemoglobin (hemoglobin A) and 80 percent is a fetal hemoglobin (hemoglobin F). Hemoglobin F persists in the infant for the first seven months of life. The same hemoglobin F has also been found in the blood of patients suffering from thalassemia, an anemia with a high incidence in regions surrounding the Mediterranean Sea. Hemoglobin F contains, as does hemoglobin A, two α-chains; the two β-chains, however, have been replaced by two quite different γ-chains. When the technique of electrophoresis was first applied to the hemoglobin of blacks suffering from sickle cell anemia in 1949, a new hemoglobin (hemoglobin S) was discovered. More than 200 different human hemoglobins have been discovered since. They differ from normal hemoglobin A in the amino acid composition of either the α- or the β-chain.

The hemoglobins of some of the lowest fishes are monomers containing one iron atom per molecule. Hemoglobin-like respiratory proteins have been found in some invertebrates. The red hemoglobin of insects, mollusks, and protozoans is called erythrocruorin. It differs from vertebrate hemoglobin by its high molecular weight.

Although green plants contain no hemoglobin, a red protein, called leghemoglobin, has been discovered in the root nodules of leguminous plants. It seems to be produced by the nitrogen-fixing bacteria of the root nodules and may be involved in the reduction of atmospheric nitrogen to ammonia and amino acids.